THE ENERGY & ART OF RESTORATIVE YOGA

ALIGNING YOUR LIFE THROUGH ENERGY WORK AND PROFOUND RELAXATION

EMILY KANE

FALLON PUBLISHING

CONTENTS

About The Energy & Art of Restorative Yoga	vii
Praise For Emily	ix
The Energy & Art of Restorative Yoga	xi
Introduction	xiii
1. Intention of Restorative Yoga	1
2. Meditation	25
3. Pranayama	31
4. Restorative Props	47
5. Injuries, Illness, and Radical Transformation	55
6. Not Being a Spiritual Asshole	64
7. Chakra Road Map	74
8. Muladhara	80
9. Svadhisthana	89
10. Manipura	99
11. Anahata	108
12. Vishuddha	119
13. Ajna	130
14. Sahasrara	140
15. Restorative Postures	150
16. Putting it all together	216
Epilogue	225
About The Author	229
References	231

Dedications and Contributors

I dedicate this book to my students, family, and friends—those who have stood by me and provided valuable teachings. To my husband, Kevin, who's love and support has helped me hold space for myself and in turn, share that gift with others.

ABOUT THE ENERGY & ART OF RESTORATIVE YOGA

"The Energy and Art of Restorative Yoga" is the ultimate guide to aligning your life with energetic work and profound relaxation. This resource explains how to apply spiritual teachings to restorative yoga, a practice built on the art of "slowing down."

This practical step-by-step guide includes valuable approaches, anecdotes, and mindsets to enhance your yoga practice and uplift your spirit. More than just a teaching resource, "The Energy and Art of Restorative Yoga" will make you rethink your outlook on life and how you live it.

PRAISE FOR EMILY

"Emily has a statuesque presence that fills the room with radiant energy. She radiates gold."

Ana Forrest - Medicine Woman, Author, and Creatrix of Forrest Yoga. Recognized worldwide as a pioneer of yoga and emotional healing.

"Emily is one of my favorite yoga teachers. I love her restorative classes and how she holds space. Her knowledge and presence are major assets to be inspired by."

Andrea Nacey – International Yoga Teacher and Owner of Cayoosh Yoga Studio

THE ENERGY & ART OF RESTORATIVE YOGA

INTRODUCTION

"Emily, you are a fuck up."

My sister sat there next to my mom with her jaw wide open, "MOM," she gasped.

Everyone was quiet. It didn't matter that it was because I forgot to take out the garbage. It could have been anything, really. That masters program I didn't get into, that time I missed a deadline, or when I burned something on the stove. It didn't matter that I had been an honours student, an award recipient, a university graduate, and a successful entrepreneur.

I know I'm not a fuck up—I am smart, funny, caring, kind, ambitious, and driven. I know that my mom loves me and wants the absolute best for me. I know that those words just slipped out of her in anger. We're all human and we all make mistakes, right? And yet, these are the messages we're fed by society every day—in advertisements, in the workplace, at home, and throughout life. We're never skinny enough, attractive enough, smart enough, spiritual enough, fit enough, or good enough. We're all just one mistake away from being a "fuck up."

Hearing these words coming out of my mother's mouth, I realized that this moment was a wake-up call. The universe was sending me a signal to make me aware of my true purpose in life. This realization identified the importance of self-love so that I could stop playing small and teach others to do the same. Part of connecting to my highest calling would be to empower those seeking belonging to be themselves instead. By lifting the burden from what weighed them down, they could be unapologetic about who they were. It would be my mission in life, somehow, to make everyone realize that they are "enough."

This is the magic of practicing restorative, a form of yoga that anyone can do. A place where no one feels "lesser than" and instead, a loving relationship with themselves is formed or strengthened. The best news is, if you have a body with some form of conscious control, then restorative yoga is accessible to you. When I found restorative yoga, it was challenging—my body and mind were not on board with being still. Slowing down was far from my default. Being athletic, determined, and ambitious kept me kicked into high gear constantly.

When I started to experience the deeper shifts that come with practicing restorative yoga, my mat became pure bliss—it was the exact medicine for the life I chose to live. The teachings of this book will provide deep healing to anyone with an intense, demanding, or stressful lifestyle. This includes anyone who identifies as an athlete, thought leader, parent, or entrepreneur. The career-driven individuals or those who are always striving for greatness will receive the most out of this approach to yoga, given that they are ready to embrace the philosophy behind the practice.

The teachings will also be invaluable for students with acute or chronic illness or injury—restorative yoga is meant to be an inclusive practice for anyone. One of my restorative yoga teachers uses a wheelchair which has never stopped her from getting on her mat. If you have bodily autonomy, in any capacity, then I am confident that restorative yoga is for you.

1

INTENTION OF RESTORATIVE YOGA
CHALLENGING YOURSELF VS. LETTING GO—FOR LIFE ON AND OFF THE MAT

One thing a lot of people get confused about with regards to "being enough" is the thought that "well, if I'm already enough, why try?" The practice of restorative yoga and loving yourself is far from complacent or lazy. In fact, I'm encouraging you to seek out your passions, reach your goals, and follow your dreams. The difference is the mentality that drives you: whether it comes from a place of intensity, fear, and loathing or kindness, compassion, and inner strength. Anyone who's overcome obstacles via both paths knows on a soul level that there's a vast difference between these motivations. Louise Hay, an inspirational author and soulful teacher, says every choice we make is either an act of self-love or self-hate.

Although it's an intense statement, the message is accurate. Intention is key when it comes to embracing self-love. There are always two ways to approach the same situation.

Running is a great example. The reason behind why someone chooses to run can come from either side of the spectrum. It can be:

- An act of self-hate: loathing or punishment to the body, penalty for overeating, and so on, or

- An act of self-love: a moving meditation, health, strength, and an endorphin rush.

The practice of restorative yoga is pure self-love when intention, presence, and surrender are involved. Slowing down is the cure to a life stuck in overdrive. This is where the lesson of "challenging yourself" vs. "letting go" comes into play. To challenge yourself in this context involves taming a rebellious mind. The mind loves finding distractions to focus on. These distractions can either be external or internal.

External distractions consist of anything happening in an immediate environment that can be picked up on by your senses—including sounds, lights, or movement. In the eight limbs of yoga, pratyahara is the practice of withdrawing the senses; this encourages the elimination of external distractions. Practicing with eyes closed is a brilliant way to practice pratyahara since it tunes out any visual distractions.

After limiting external interruptions, the next layer is revealed—the interferences that come with thoughts and emotions, or internal distractions. Meditation is the solution to counteract internal distractions. Dharana is known as meditative concentration, which is developed by attaining a clear focus using meditation techniques to calm the fluctuations of the mind, including thoughts and emotions. Ultimately, challenging yourself requires action to reduce these external and internal distractions.

Letting go, on the other hand, demands a deep sense of honesty and trust when it comes to expectations. One of the aspects of restorative yoga that I absolutely love is that it asks you to "do less" which is extremely difficult if you're accustomed to working at 150%. This means that, even if you "can" do something, you consciously choose to practice differently to create ease.

That might mean taking a variation, using more props, or practicing a completely different posture. A metaphor for this action of "doing less" would be the difference between taking a shower and a bubble bath. Sure, they both get you clean, but taking a bubble bath can be relaxing, indulgent, and nourishing. The intention of the restorative practice is to find those illuminating qualities throughout your time on your mat.

Rather than staying in a restorative posture that's just "ok," you position your body to experience luxurious relaxation. Embodying these characteristics can be as simple as using more props to support yourself, applying the props differently, or taking a different posture altogether. This can be terrifying for some students, especially if adhering to directions and orders are part of a habitual pattern.

Many of us have internalized these patterns from childhood. Parents, teachers, coaches, and other leaders have instilled these beliefs within children, so that they'll always listen to authority figures. This is great in childhood when structure propels their learning. It also fosters a deep respect for others, including their elders.

The issue happens when those children grow into adults that have difficulty using keen discernment when taking direction from anyone in a place of power. Yoga teachers are viewed as "experts" in their field, which makes them an authority figure on the subject in the eyes of the student.

This leads some students to give over their personal power—choosing to listen solely to the instructions of the teacher while ignoring valid messages that their body is offering them. This pattern of listening to authority while excluding personal needs is a pattern that must be broken if a student seeks any kind of growth.

Letting go of expectations, of the self and that of the teacher, is the path to creating freedom by expressing your truth. Nurturing this confidence when practicing restorative yoga is bound to be a catalyst for positive change.

RESTORATIVE YOGA WITH A CAPITAL "R"

Over the years, I've noticed a shift in the restorative styles offered in public yoga classes. Just like hatha and vinyasa, the essence of restorative yoga has expanded to include a broader scope. Seeing this emergence of varying styles of restorative has its benefits, however, it can be confusing when choosing a class and a teacher. Being clear on the style of restorative yoga offered is key.

My friend and colleague, Maeve Jones, refers to the most relaxing, supported, and meditative styles as "restorative yoga with a capital R." To me, this makes perfect sense: the capital "R" symbolizes the importance of putting restoration first. This definition recognizes that there are multiple restorative styles, leaving restorative yoga with a capital "R" at the very far end of the spectrum, indicating the most relaxing, supported, and comfortable decision for postures offered.

To clarify, there is a difference between *practicing a pose in a restorative way* and *practicing restorative yoga.* Practicing a yoga posture in a restorative way suggests taking a more active variation from a hatha tradition—either seated or laying down—and encouraging a more passive stretch. For example, relaxing your legs and the muscles around your spine during a forward fold would be more restorative than maintaining a contraction. Although this can have therapeutic benefits, I would caution against calling it "restorative yoga." Practicing postures in a restorative way is aligned with gentle hatha and yin yoga, which are both wonderful, but the intention is quite different from restorative yoga with a capital "R."

In recent years, it's become apparent that there is some confusion between restorative and yin yoga. Both are relaxing, passive styles of yoga which visually, appear very similar. Despite their initial appearance, each style has a unique intention to experience as a practitioner. Yin yoga is an ideal practice for anyone with excessive tension, especially athletes.

Despite how relaxing yin yoga can be, it still has a very different purpose to restorative yoga. The practice seeks to lean into strong sensations, which is meant to release the deeper connective tissues in the body, mainly the fascia.

Ultimately, this means pursuing a deeper stretch with longer holds. Although props can be used, they are not essential to the yin yoga practice. Restorative yoga, on the other hand, seeks very subtle sensations and uses an abundance of props. This emphasizes a completely relaxed and supported state. This complete support with the use of props signals to the nervous system to fully relax which is extremely powerful.

Although yin yoga offers some nervous system regulation, it does not compare with the effects of restorative yoga with a capital "R." The consistency of deep relaxation is what makes it unique. The profound impact that restorative has on the nervous system cannot be matched by any other style of asana practice.

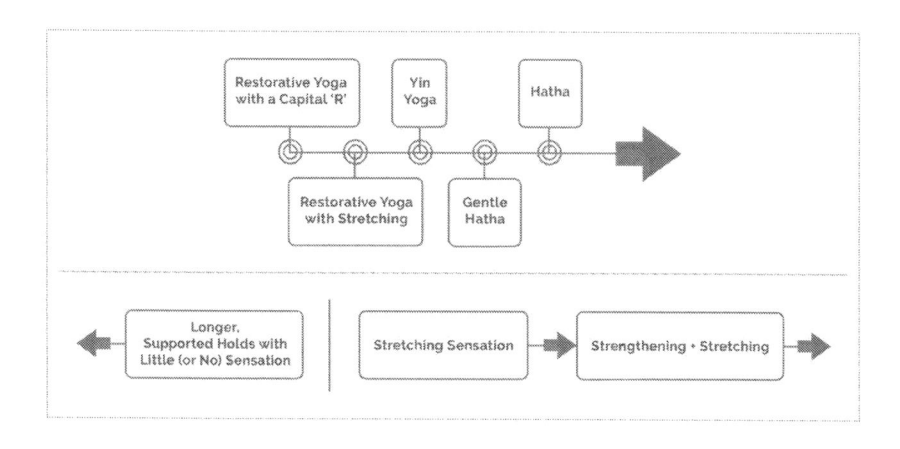

THE FOUR GUIDELINES FOR RESTORATIVE YOGA WITH A CAPITAL "R":

1. Focus on Subtle Sensations

For the A-Type perfectionists, this will be by far the most challenging concept to grasp. For those accustomed to "playing through the pain" or "feeling the burn," it will be hard to focus on doing less. For many yoga practitioners, having the absence of strong stretching sensations may even feel unsettling at first. The common reactions are "am I doing this right?" or "will I see a benefit if I don't feel a stretch?"

The significance of "doing less" is not just about what there is to gain, but instead asking "what is there to lose?"

Following this guideline naturally holds space to let go of self-doubt, self-sabotage, poor self-esteem, and negative body image. Creating space to evolve by letting go of limiting patterns is an essential part of the healing process. An example would be to make decisions unapologetically about the postures and variations you choose. This ensures that anything selected is an expression of self-love, compassion, and understanding.

Something to keep in mind that has helped me over the years: the ego loves deep, juicy, intense sensations but the soul loves relaxation and restorative yoga. Be mindful of how your intention and energy supports your healing.

2. Stay in postures for time

"Time heals all wounds" is an appropriate saying when it comes to restorative yoga. Time is a magical thing—it gives the body an opportunity to shift physiologically from a sympathetic state, or the stress response, into the parasympathetic, or the relaxation response (aka rest and digest). This act of "letting off the gas" has biological expressions, but perhaps more importantly, it has an impact on state of mind. The mind isn't like a switch when it comes to relaxation—it needs time to unwind. A bare minimum of 3 minutes should be given to each posture. Generally, anywhere from 5 – 15 minutes works best to experience the bliss that comes with deep relaxation.

Beyond the physical benefits of staying in postures for longer, there are also advantages for emotional and spiritual well-being. In a world that often encourages us to go faster, be stronger, do better, and to always be striving for "more" it is magical to have a clear space to do less. In fact, to have no other task than to be fully present with body and breath is profoundly healing for those who struggle with these pressures on a regular basis.

3. Props, props, and more props

The idea of "less is more" is a common philosophy in restorative yoga —except when it comes to props. Approaching the practice with "the more the merrier" is the best way to sustain restorative postures. It's essential to use an abundance of props effectively in this style of practice. This firm support for the body assists the nervous system in bringing forth the relaxation response.

Props can include conventional yoga tools such as bolsters, blocks, eye pillows, and straps but non-conventional props can be integrated as well. This makes home practices very accessible since couch pillows, chairs, ottomans, and other furniture are useful too. There may be certain postures that require less props, but to have a complete restorative practice, props are a necessity.

4. Holding space for focus and stillness

Meditation and restorative yoga have similar intentions. While meditating, you're meant to be comfortable to bring focus from the physical body to the mind. That way, the practitioner becomes aware of the natural ebbs and flows of consciousness, drifting between lucid and dreamlike states. However, in restorative yoga, the postures act as the vessel for altered states of consciousness instead of being seated as in meditation.

Harnessing the mind with its fluctuations is usually the greatest obstacle. A common response is to reject or push thoughts away, however, it is empowering to accept that thoughts naturally come up. Realistically, thinking is what the mind is programmed to do! Struggling with the thoughts that pop up only creates more resistance, making it impossible to surrender. The best route asks practitioners to act with compassion and understanding.

Finding a point of focus is a game-changer in those moments when thoughts or emotions are running wild. "Catching" oneself during those times is a strong lesson. Picking up the pieces and starting over is a skill everyone must learn, especially in a meditative style of practice, which is ultimately a metaphor for life itself. Eventually, with time and patience, the mind switches gears and accepts stillness. Shifting between these two states of focus and stillness creates space for learning, growth, and insight.

THE NERVOUS SYSTEM AND RESTORATIVE YOGA

Nervous system regulation is an essential benefit of restorative yoga. For those who grapple with stress daily, restorative yoga is the ultimate therapeutic approach. With a culture that prioritizes high expectations and fast technology, practicing restorative yoga becomes an integral part of physical, mental, emotional, and spiritual health.

The nervous system and its regulation impacts us on all levels. It's no coincidence that those with high levels of cortisol (stress hormone) experience higher levels of depression, anxiety, fatigue, and chronic illness. The inherent principles of restorative yoga are meant to reinforce the healing of the nervous system.

Understanding relaxation starts with grasping the divisions of the nervous system that are broken down into the structural and functional divisions. The structural division is made up of the brain and spinal cord which is considered the central nervous system (CNS). The peripheral nervous system includes the cranial and spinal nerves so that the brain can communicate via the spinal cord with the rest of the body.

This links with the motor (efferent) division through nerve impulses from the CNS to the effectors aka muscles and glands. The two branches of the motor division are the somatic nervous system, which we control like skeletal muscle, and the autonomic nervous system (ANS) which—arguably—is not in our control. Although it is universally accepted that the reaction of the ANS is completely automatic, more progressive perspectives suggest that our mental and emotional health has a significant influence on how this system functions.

More specifically, the response to potential stressors impacting how the nervous system integrates sensory information, meaning that if we perceive an event to be stressful, the nervous system will react accordingly, versus when we don't recognize the same situation as a threat. Shifting perspective mentally and emotionally can greatly influence how the ANS responds to any event.

In terms of sensory input, information brought through the ANS will affect glands that impact cardiac and smooth muscle. The adrenal glands hold significance in restorative yoga since they produce various hormones in response to stress. When leading an active life full of potential stressors, finding balance means decreasing the influence of stress propagated by the adrenal glands. There are two systems that have an impact on stress, including glands, known as the sympathetic and parasympathetic nervous system—both are divisions of the ANS and play a major role in restorative yoga.

The sympathetic nervous system is known as the "fight-or-flight" response and reacts during times of stress to protect against potential threats. From an evolutionary perspective, this was meant to defend oneself in life-or-death situations to ensure the survival of our species. For instance, if you came across a bear, you would need to know whether it is necessary to fight or flee in order to survive. Although this system plays an important role, problems surface when there are situations that are not threatening to our survival yet cause the same reaction, often for a prolonged and unnecessary period of time.

When this response is constantly "turned on," it leads to health issues including high blood pressure, metabolic disorders, and other diseases. On the other hand, the parasympathetic nervous system is crucial to finding deep relaxation; it acts as the "brake" while the sympathetic is the gas. Both systems are tonally active, meaning that they always provide a degree of nervous input to a given tissue.

When the parasympathetic nervous system is dominant, it assists in relieving the pressures of stress, especially when it comes to the physiological consequences. This response will decrease blood pressure, heart rate, stress hormones, and increase digestion—making it clear as to why this is referred to colloquially as the "rest-and-digest" response. Many tissues are innervated by both systems considering that the sympathetic and parasympathetic typically have opposing effects. There are a few exceptions; take the skin, sweat glands, and blood vessels, for instance. Most blood vessels in the entire body only receive sympathetic nerve fibers, so in this circumstance, a more appropriate analogy might be "gas" and "letting off the gas" rather than gas and brake.

Instead of viewing the opposing responses as "good" or "bad," it's important to understand that both play important roles regarding health and well-being. Finding balance is key, meaning that those who experience frequent stress need more parasympathetic activation on a regular basis for their health and well-being.

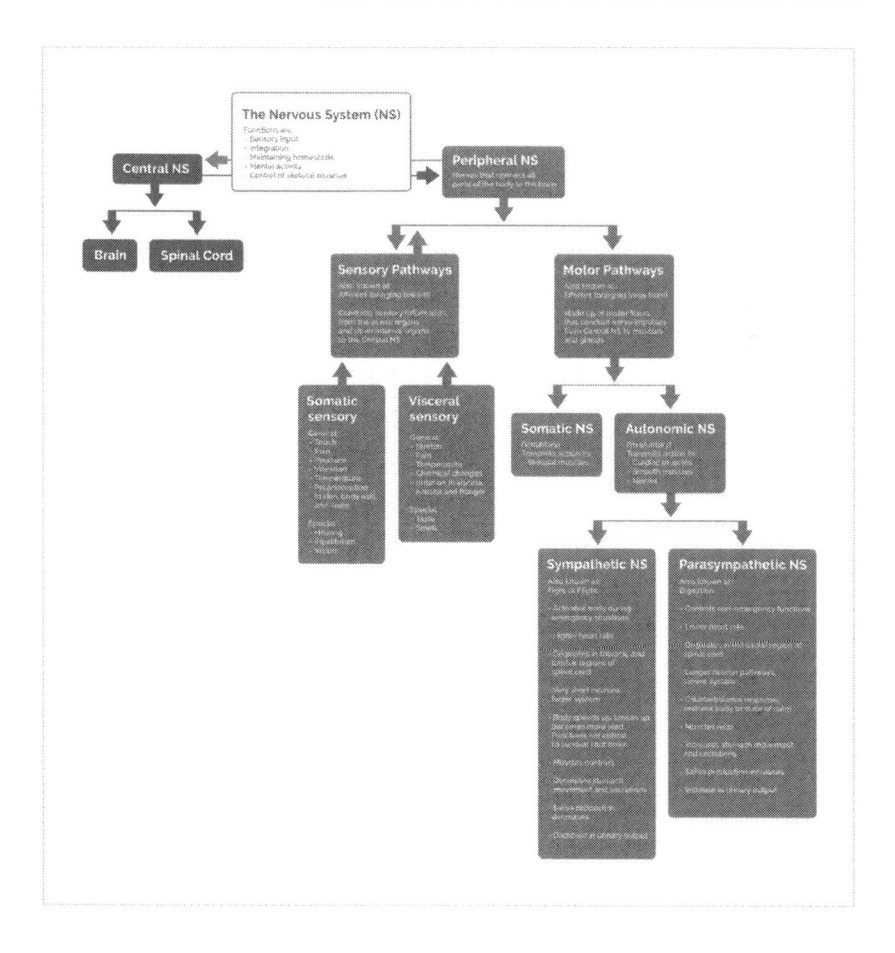

The body has sensory receptors to determine muscular length and tension, known as muscle spindles and golgi tendon organs (GTO), which assist us with proprioception—the awareness of where our body is in space. These structures prevent us from getting injured by over-stretching tissues. When tissues are being stretched, these receptors are alert to make sure that they aren't being overstretched, which can cause damage.

The theory in restorative yoga is that the autonomic nervous system still offers some sympathetic tone under these circumstances, meaning that stretching will not fully allow you to relax. Allowing yourself to experience very subtle sensations, or no sensation at all, will give the parasympathetic nervous system—or relaxation response—an opportunity to work miracles. For those coping with stress, pressure, or excessive activity, the act of complete relaxation is very therapeutic. The effects of the parasympathetic nervous system include decreases in blood pressure, heart rate, blood lactate, and more, while supporting digestion and elimination. The healing impact of the parasympathetic nervous system goes beyond the measurable reactions that happen physically. The relaxation response also produces theta brain waves, a rhythmic pattern of neural activity. This oscillation is characterized by a greater amplitude and slower frequency than alpha or beta waves which are present in an alert state.

These theta waves are the gateway to learning, memory, and intuition, so it's no surprise that this rhythm is associated with healing and expansiveness. In terms of the physiological response, theta waves share advantages with the nervous system that occur from relaxation, but they are also known to foster spiritual experiences. Increased awareness and meaningful epiphanies come with a deeper understanding of ourselves and the world—concepts that become clearer with profound relaxation. Having these spiritual experiences that arise out of theta state can help us see how our human experience is more than a physical one. This realization makes it clear that energetic presence can be just as important as the health of the body—and that the two are intrinsically connected.

ADDITIONAL BENEFITS OF RESTORATIVE YOGA

Restorative yoga boasts numerous benefits for physical health. Physiologically, the relief that comes with the parasympathetic response has repercussions on nearly every other system. For instance, Asadollahi et al looked at the impact of mindfulness and relaxation on weight loss. A widely held belief in our society exclusively links weight loss to activities with physical exertion. In this study, obese patients experienced weight loss by introducing mindfulness and meditation—both are forms of relaxation, basic tenets of restorative yoga.

On the flip side, the damage of an overactive stress response from the sympathetic nervous system increases levels of cortisol—a stress hormone released during sympathetic activation. Circulating cortisol and psychosocial stress may contribute to obesity and metabolic syndromes. Adrenaline is also released during stress, and over time, the chronic production of these two hormones stops the body from recovering—resulting in serious health problems. Chronic stress can contribute to digestive issues, a weakened immune response, cardiovascular disease, depression, anxiety, and other mood disorders. Neuroendocrine circadian rhythms—or the periodic self-sustained release of hormones—can be disrupted by stress. Numerous studies have shown that this disruption can favor the growth and metastasis of tumors. Metastasized tumors are resistant to conventional forms of therapy, making them a major cause of death from cancer. By using methods that relieve stress regularly, these chronic and acute diseases can be prevented.

Beyond disease prevention, the art of relaxation helps with aging gracefully. The brain benefits when the harmful effect of chronic stress is avoided through the aging process. The hippocampus, an area associated with learning and memory, is negatively affected by a prolonged stress response. It's even been suggested that avoiding chronic stress can prevent Alzheimer's and dementia, both associated with age-related decline.

With these benefits alone, it makes sense to prioritize conscious relaxation. The only requirement to advance or sustain your health is stepping into it with the right intention and sticking to a consistent practice—if that seems unmanageable right now, having the willingness to step onto a new path can work miracles. Every journey starts with a single step, and this might be yours. Even making just a little bit of time each day can make a difference.

STRETCHING VS. RELEASING

In restorative yoga, we practice with the intention of releasing or opening. Having this focus supports the nervous system with settling into the parasympathetic response. The sensation of stretching, or any feelings of depth or intensity, are signals to ease into a more restful position. This can be done one of two ways, either by using additional props or coming out of the posture altogether. It's better to be lying face up or down while relaxed instead of struggling in an uncomfortable shape.

Most of us are so accustomed to suffering—at our work, in our homes, and in school—taking on stress and tension has become the norm in our fast-paced culture. Saying "yes" to relaxation and being able to surrender fully is one of the few opportunities there are to embrace comfort without any guilt.

Students who are new to restorative often find this notion of releasing or opening—rather than stretching—a difficult concept to grasp. Although there are benefits to stronger stretching sensations in a hatha, vinyasa, or a yin yoga practice, the intention of restorative is to attain depth in the response from the nervous system. "Doing less" makes it possible to receive the subtle benefits which tends to be tough for anyone who is ambitious, driven, and physically active.

Often, it's the exact medicine these individuals require to heal. Slowing down to do less is rarely in the vocabulary of achieving go-getters with high standards and a packed schedule. From this point of view, stretching is seen as accomplishing a task, whereas lacking sensation is a foreign concept. To recognize the benefits of exploring deep relaxation through prolonged comfort will shift that perspective. For instance, the act of practicing active yoga or sitting quietly in meditations will have varying outcomes on health. Although both are beneficial, you will see different results from committing to one over the other.

Focusing on the subtle sensations takes the emphasis away from the physical, which shifts the attention to the mental, emotional, and energetic aspects of the practice. Physical phenomena become less of a priority since body and breath are a gateway to a deeper experience.

Stretching is not "bad," rather the priority shifts to a different intention in restorative yoga, one that favours comfort and ease to foster a meditative state. Although a subtle stretch is appropriate, in this case referring to a release or opening, feelings of intensity should be avoided to fully experience the healing impact of this therapeutic practice. To open yourself up to the possibilities associated with restorative yoga, one must be willing to be completely honest with themselves about the sensations they are experiencing. Furthermore, when these perceptions do arise, it is essential to act swiftly. Taking action is as simple as adding more props or easing out of the posture to take a different variation altogether. Gaining the courage and confidence to recognize these moments of power is one of the gifts that is cultivated by this style of practice. With enough repetition, these traits begin to trickle into everyday life.

TIPS FOR PRACTICING

What to wear:

Any clothing that is comfortable and does not restrict movement is perfect for restorative yoga. Body-hugging athleisure is completely optional as is loose-fitting clothing. The body's temperature may drop during longer sequences since there's very little movement involved, so it is worthwhile to have a sweater, warm socks, or an extra blanket, especially if you are prone to getting cold.

Timing:

Timing can be a challenge with restorative yoga—time seems altered when it's slowed down through long supported holds; most postures seem to fly by in an instant. Using a timer is highly recommended to keep the focus on remaining in a meditative state rather than questioning how long the posture has lasted. If you are using a timer on your phone or tablet, check that the device isn't sending or receiving signals (i.e. airplane mode with the WiFi turned off) to ensure a distraction-free practice.

What if there's not enough time?

Even practicing 5 or 10 minutes of savasana is better than nothing. Start small and fit it in when you can. There are some postures that you can practice anywhere, at any time. Take meditation for example; you can apply the techniques while standing in line for groceries or waiting on a bus. If your mindset is present, it's a chance to connect with your body and breath. For your home practice, even setting aside small chunks of time in a day can do wonders.

Distractions:

These days, there's always something! Whether you have kids, pets, loud neighbors, or construction outside… the list can be endless. Rather than get caught up in what can't be controlled, focus on what can be done to set the tone for your practice. This includes:

- Setting clear boundaries with those who live with you. This may include you/them moving to another room.
- Remove any unnecessary distractions including light or noise where possible.
- Finally, (and most importantly) embrace the distractions that can't be controlled. These too are blessings meant to challenge us so that we can grow! In these moments, a sense of humour can be our greatest ally. A little laughter is good for the soul.

Before Practicing:

- Do your best to avoid eating a couple of hours before. If that is not avoidable, eat very lightly, like a smoothie or a piece of

fruit. Digesting can create agitation so it's best to practice on an empty stomach.
- Organize your props by choosing the postures you'd like to practice with the recommendations provided
- Set the tone. This might mean dimming lights, using essential oils, or playing soothing background music.

Contraindications:

For many health concerns and injuries, there are certain postures that will feel amazing while others should be avoided. There can be two students with the same condition that experience different symptoms regarding pain. This means that even though both are managing "X," one posture is appropriate for one student but not the other. The true answer to whether a posture is suitable to practice is "it depends," since the severity and experience of the condition can vary greatly from person to person.

Each student has a right to bodily autonomy, determining what movements or positions may exacerbate a condition or cause pain. Although there are recommendations that highlight "proceeding with caution," know that this list is not definitive. If you have a health condition and are unsure whether a posture is right for you, discuss with your doctor, physiotherapist, or a medical professional.

> **Note:** Although restorative yoga can be accessible to all, it is not a replacement for medical treatment.

This book resource is meant to supplement your health, not replace medical interventions. Please discuss with a health care professional to find the right variations that will fit with your condition.

One condition that has caused a controversial stir in the yoga community is menstruation. The questions of "should I" or "should I not" with certain postures during this time has mixed opinions from experienced yoga teachers, especially for inversions. Rumours have circulated stressing the potential physiological consequences, luckily none of which has been scientifically proven.

However, that does not mean there is no merit to avoiding certain postures during menstruation. The energetic consequences should also be considered for women since it is possible to support our body's natural frequency. The notion of "prana" and "apana" is of great significance in these circumstances. Prana, or life force energy, has five vayus, or "winds." Prana vayu is related to life force energy, typically associated with inward moving energy, to nourish our systems, while apana is linked to the outward moving energy, or the body's need to release what it is no longer using.

Naturally, the prana vayu is activated with our inhale and apana comes with the exhale. Food is another example; prana is taken in by the meals we eat while apana exits the body as waste. Menstruation illustrates the action of apana as it's released from the body. To facilitate this process energetically, it's only natural to be in positions that allow the unobstructed flow of a menstrual cycle to occur. This means, avoiding tilting the uterus in a direction that prevents this flow, as happens during inversions. In a relaxed position, even a slight posterior (backwards) tilt can cause discomfort when the hips are raised up above the heart. Although each woman has the right to choose what will work for her body, the energetic role of apana stands as an important consideration.

Finding the "right" fit for you with variations in your practice is possible with curiosity, your body's innate wisdom, and with supportive health care providers. Adding a new prop or using one in a new way can bring up bliss that was never thought possible. Why settle for "just ok" when luxury is just one blanket or block away! Exploring is part of the experience in restorative yoga and you're about to receive your map.

Is there a "right way" and a "wrong way" to practice?

"Thank you for correcting me," is a comment I've received from multiple students over the years. On a similar tangent, the question, "am I doing this right?" also comes up. In yoga, there are so many different perspectives. Even in science, new research is released daily. Our view on movement shifts over time as new viewpoints emerge. There's a very dominant, fiery energy that wants to "be right" and know the correct answer to be validated. The truth is, what is "right" is based on your experience rather than what someone else tells you to do.

No one has ever lived a minute in your body. So how can someone else have a better opinion on your experience? If there is any concern about whether the practice is being done "right," the more important question is "am I coming back to the intention of this practice?" If you are relaxing, present, and surrendering, you're doing exactly what you need to do. Even if you aren't "quite there" mentally, if you are trying your best to arrive, then that is perfect! Focusing on how your physical body feels—rather than on how it looks—will tell you everything you need to know.

Everything provided in this book is a suggestion based on my experiences and what I've noticed with students. Your experience may be different and there's absolutely nothing wrong with that. Take everything offered as an invitation, instead of a command, and open yourself to the possibilities.

One last concept that proves helpful comes from the yoga sutras: "sthira sukham asanam," translating to: every asana (pose) is steady, stable, and comfortable. If a restorative posture resonates with this intention, then by yoga philosophy's standards, you are perfect. When you can't get a certain posture to fit this intention, then you have permission to change the shape—perhaps more props—or even to practice a completely different posture. It's that simple. You are empowered to make the call, so use your power wisely.

BREATH

Breath is a powerful tool. Without breathing, we would cease to exist, making it necessary for our survival and even spiritual development. Inhalations and exhalations maintain an exchange of oxygen and carbon dioxide essential for life itself. On a more subtle level, prana—life force energy—is brought in on an inhalation, while apana—what's often described as a downward and outward flow of energy—is carried out during exhalation. The muscle that makes these exchanges possible is the diaphragm, located just beneath the ribcage.

The specific attachment points are the xiphoid process at the base of the sternum, the costal cartilages of the lower six ribs, and the first three lumbar vertebrae. This is important since certain asana change the shape of these bones, potentially altering the level of functioning for the diaphragm.

The facet joints of the thoracic and lumbar vertebrae play a part in the movement of the diaphragm. Quality of breathing is affected by the mobility of these joints that tend to be influenced by spinal extension—often referred to as "back-bending" postures like a sphynx or supported bridge. One of the fascinating fascial connections with the diaphragm is with the psoas—a major hip flexor. This muscle joins the trunk to the legs and is known for assisting with locomotion.

It is also a major muscle affected by the "fight or flight" response. Back when humans were hunters and gatherers, this stress response prepared us to fight or flee in life-or-death situations. This response from the autonomic nervous system protected us in serious situations.

If you encountered a bear attack while gathering, would you really have time to think and prepare? This meant that the muscles for running or fighting would need to be ready to go. Enter the psoas, a powerhouse muscle that could be ready for anything. Unfortunately for those with chronic stress, tightness in the psoas is likely an unnecessary repercussion. The fascial connection of the diaphragm and psoas suggests that releasing tension in the psoas may lead to better breathing.

The movement of the diaphragm that regulates breathing might seem confusing at first but makes complete sense upon closer inspection. With an inhalation, the abdominal cavity expands, but this expansion is associated with the lungs—not expansion of the diaphragm.

For the lungs to expand, the diaphragm needs to flatten, or contract, to decrease the pressure in the lungs. Air always moves from areas of high to low pressure. This decrease in pressure allows outside air to enter the lungs, causing an increase in pressure resulting in the expansion of the ribs and abdomen. During exhalation is when the diaphragm relaxes; it expands to return to its dome-like shape. This action of breathing is assisted by the intercostals as well as the elastic recoil of the lungs and ribs.

An interesting fact about the mechanism of breathing comes from this question: why do we breathe in the first place? Most people would answer "because we need oxygen." To that I would say yes, we do need oxygen, but this isn't what prompts our body to breathe. If that has you raising any eyebrows, bear with me. To understand why we breathe, we need to understand hyperventilation.

Hyperventilation is not caused by the need for more oxygen, it is triggered by an imbalance of carbon dioxide. Read that again. With gasping inhales, the act of hyperventilating looks that way at first. However, consider "the cure" for hyperventilation. Have you ever seen a movie where a kid is breathing into a paper bag? The bag is inflating and deflating but it's just a paper bag!

And it's certainly not oxygen. They are increasing the amount of carbon dioxide in the paper bag in order to find balance. By increasing the amount of carbon dioxide in their system, they stop hyperventilating. Thus, our body is not seeking ways to get more oxygen—it is prompted to breathe by high levels of carbon dioxide. It is interesting to see how exhales can be labelled negatively as "toxic" or "waste," when having a certain concentration is just as important as the oxygen we breathe in.

Even physiology can be a reminder that the world is not black or white—or "good" and "bad"—that at the end of the day, balance is key. Seeing both the black and the white—or in this case, the inhale and the exhale—as essential to our existence is part of understanding that delicate balance.

When it comes to the balancing act of breathing applied to a yoga practice, it's easy to get caught up in the details. One question students have is "when should I breathe?" In other words, when should I inhale and exhale? Typically, an inhale is meant to be lengthening, lifting, or expansive, whereas an exhale is appropriate for actions relating to closing off, reducing, or lowering. "Closing off" in this context refers to making one area of the body smaller—like in flexion for example.

The name of the game is "feeling" rather than overthinking. There will be certain places where it feels natural to inhale or exhale. Drop the logic to favor your intuition. It will always give you the right answer. If you're not sure, try both and pick one based on what you feel. On the topic of intuition, this skill can be used for more than just when to breathe. It can be applied to how you'd like breath to flow intentionally.

The act of breathing into your pelvis or sending breath down into your feet may seem ridiculous, "but Emily, I don't have lungs in my feet!" Of course, you don't. But rather than take this literally, see it as an opportunity to come back to intention. Intention being: can this breath be used to create space so that this area releases, either physically or spiritually? Bringing awareness using breath can create physical sensations of letting go in the tissues but there is also an energetic impact.

Think of your breath as a vessel for spiritual surgery. It has the potential to go into those areas to wash out the energetic residue that doesn't need to be stored there anymore. By breathing directly into these "spots," we use prana to break up what no longer serves the body or the spirit—holding space so that we can embrace health and freedom.

BODY SCAN

A body scan will enhance the experience of each posture every time you settle in. This routine indicates where your body is still holding onto tension, even if you're not initially aware of it. Often there are unconscious patterns of holding that can only be released when we become aware of their presence. Cultivating awareness using a body scan, from your toes up through your body all the way to your head, can be used to encourage complete relaxation. Here is an example of a body scan, step by step:

- Relax through your toes and ankles, let your heels get heavier
- Soften through the backs of your legs, allow your pelvis to sink deeper into the mat
- Relax the muscles around your spine
- Let shoulders relax away from ears and into your mat
- Arms and the backs of your hands get heavier
- Feel the length along the back of your neck, soften through your throat
- Let the back of your head release into the mat
- Soften any tension in your face—forehead, jaw, and the space between your eyebrows
- Let that relaxation flow into your breath

The interesting part about a body scan is that it will be different every time you practice it. Different postures will influence what you feel, not to mention changes from day-to-day life, activities, and stressors. Going through a body scan methodically in each posture builds focus, which is beneficial for meditation and relaxation.

It also creates an awareness of where we can "breathe" into. For every shape, there is a slightly different area that breath gravitates towards. In certain postures, you may feel spaciousness in your back, others in your belly or chest. This largely depends on form—for instance, if the belly is restricted from folding forward, then breath will naturally fill the back.

Alternatively, a side opening may emphasize movement in the ribcage along the side of the body. This is your chance to develop a curiosity about where breath naturally flows to. There's no "right" or "wrong" answer, given that your breath is flowing easefully without restriction or strain. Let go of the need to get it "right" and tap into what is perfect for you.

2

MEDITATION

THE MINDSET AND TOOLS OF RESTORATIVE YOGA

Meditation and restorative yoga are not so different. In fact, when you consider the basic "rules" at the heart of these practices, restorative yoga might as well be meditation with postures. Meditating requires you to be physically relaxed to focus. Pillows and other forms of support are used to make sitting comfortable, taking attention away from the body so it doesn't act as a distraction for the mind.

It's common for new meditators to get irritated when they start their practice. Even experienced meditators have days when their mind bucks like a wild horse. Getting into the "flow" can take time and conscious effort but even on the tough days it's not impossible with a few tools in your toolbox. Having these meditative skills are an asset to your restorative practice. Keeping the mind peaceful will enhance the nervous system and vice versa—a blissful feedback loop that can be accessed directly through meditation.

So, what do these "tools" of meditation look like? These are techniques to support you in getting into and staying in that meditative flow. First, we need to look into how this is accomplished in the first place. To understand the flow, we need to recognize the relationship between Dharana—meditative concentration—and Dhyana—meditative absorption. Although the two concepts seem similar, the meditative experience is a balancing act between the two. The first, Dharana, uses a point of focus to get into meditative flow.

This point of focus or "concentration" is a technique that uses mantra, images, breath, or bodily sensations to help get you into a state of flow. Once you're in that stream of consciousness, it's considered a shift into Dhyana. "Absorption" suggests being fully immersed in the experience without any point of focus. When Dhyana is present, there's no thought, only a clear stream of consciousness.

The minute that a thought pops up, you're out of that flow (Dhyana), signaling the need to jump back to a point of focus or Dharana. This flux between Dharana and Dhyana is the whole ebb and flow that makes up the meditative practice. This dance between conscious awareness and pure consciousness reminds us that meditation is not "thinking about nothing" all the time.

In fact, the original purpose of meditation was not to clear the mind at all. The fundamental basis of the practice was to liberate us from suffering. Attachment is considered one of the root causes of suffering —in this case, attaching to thoughts. According to buddha, attachment is the desire to have and not to have—also known as craving and aversion. When we can't satisfy what we crave—or when we can't escape the things we don't want—we get frustrated and angry which results in suffering.

Allowing the mind to run wild "attaching" itself to random stories will perpetuate this cycle of misery. How many stories have we told ourselves that are actually "real" and how many are just projections of our experiences? Perhaps we've slapped a few labels on an experience as "good" or "bad" or even rehashed it to consider multiple scenarios —all constructed by our imagination.

Whether these are thoughts rooted in the past or predictions piecing together what the future holds, most of it has no real stake in what's happening right now. All we have is the present—happening continuously as we live and breathe. To simmer down these fluctuations means addressing the attachment to the thoughts that are building these stories that take us out of the present. Our salvation is in controlling the mind by finding focus to create a steady stream of consciousness.

With enough practice, this flow can result in creating pure bliss known as "Samadhi." In meditation, the clearing of the mind is more of a side effect rather than the objective, with the true purpose being to find freedom and bliss. Discovering freedom and bliss starts with having a stable base of support or what's known as sthira sukham asanam—the yoga sutra confirming that every posture should be steady, stable, and comfortable. If you are practicing in a seated meditation here are a few suggestions:

SUKAHSANA (EASY POSE)

Although sukahsana is the most common posture for meditation, don't feel that your practice is limited to just seated. Meditation can be done in alternate sitting positions—kneeling or with your back against a wall for example—as well as standing or even walking. If you are fully present and focused, you are practicing meditation. The following techniques are invaluable for seated meditation but can also be directly applied to postures during a restorative sequence.

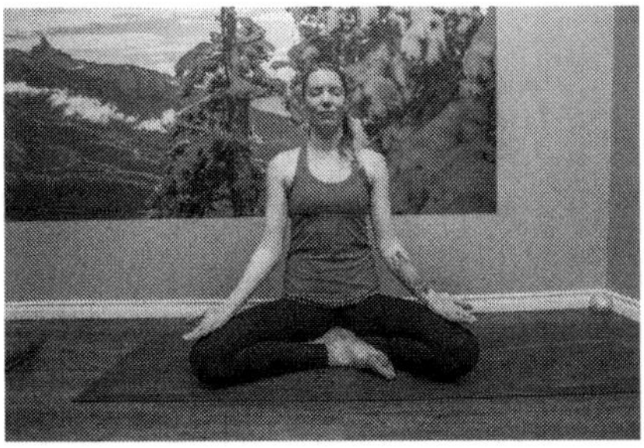

Fig. 2.1

Breath and Bodily Awareness

This is likely the most widely used technique for meditation, using the body and breath as a point of focus. The "body scan" is a form of meditation. Using different points in sequence, from the feet all the way up the head, you can start to relax those places that might still be gripping or unconsciously tight. Then, you shift that awareness to your breath. It is so fascinating once you start to get curious about your breath. You can feel your breath passing in and out through your nose or witness the cool of your inhale and the warmth of your exhale. Even how your breath creates movement in your body becomes captivating—the widening of the belly and ribcage with the lift of the collarbones. Following your breath and its characteristics can keep you focused—in a state of Dharana—so that you can shift into Dhyana more easefully.

Imagery

If you consider yourself a visual person, using imagery in your meditation can be extremely helpful. Visualizations are the most powerful when the place you send yourself to is one that brings you peace. As a snowboarder, I love visualizing being in the mountains—it's a place I feel safe and relaxed. You might find that being in the woods, on a beach, or next to a lake might work better for you. There's no limit to your imagination given that this is a place that invokes bliss and that you invite your breath to stay steady.

If thoughts become persistent, you can use imagery to package them up in a bubble or cloud, then watch them float away in the sky. Then, come back to your breath. If another thought pops up, repeat the visualization.

Mantra

A mantra is defined as a word or sound that is said repeatedly, either out loud or in the mind, to aid in concentration. A meditation could be doing ten rounds of "Om"—the universal vibration—repeated out loud or it in your head with every exhale. Repeating a set of words or affirmations in your head can be a great way to meditate, especially when it's connected with breath.

An example would be "inhaling I am peaceful, exhaling I am free" or one from Thich Nhat Hanh would be "inhaling I calm my body, exhaling I smile." If there's something that you want to cultivate in your life, you can call that in through a mantra. For instance, if you want to nurture abundance, the mantra could look like: "I am abundance" (on inhale) and "I attract everything I need" (with the exhale). Or, to keep it simple, think "love" on your inhale and "light" on your exhale, which can be paired easily with imagery.

Avoid using mantras that involve things you don't want, keep the focus on what you want to lean into rather than what you don't. You may wonder "…but what if I don't want something? Wouldn't I want to say, "I don't want to be ____ anymore." Although this seems like a natural step to "call in what you want", it does the opposite. By saying "I don't want ____" you are manifesting more of that "thing" you don't want to let into your life. Think of it like this: if I say "don't think about purple elephants", what's the first thing you think of? Purple elephants.

Manifestation works in the same manner. Therefore, when working with mantras we always want to put intention on what we want to cultivate instead of the things we need to clear out.

A WORD ON "OM"

Someone once told me they thought chanting "Om" was disturbing. This was heartbreaking to hear! It was clear this person did not understand the roots of this auspicious and comforting mantra. This healing vibration is like coming home. It is not meant to be religious —although some perceive it that way—perhaps because it was the sound that was present when the universe began. A sound that still ripples throughout the universe, resonating at the frequency in which everything exists.

Take a look around you right now—that table, or that couch, that tree, or that blade of grass—everything on a cellular level is buzzing and colliding. Science tells us that even the most "perceived" solid material is moving on an atomic level. What we recognize as mass, liquid, or gas is just a series of atoms bumping into each other. All matter vibrates at the frequency of "Om" including the cells that make up our body. It is in this way that we are completely in tune with the universe.

You could even say we are one with everything outside of ourselves, considering we are made up of the same matter that created the moon, the sky, and the stars. This vibration of "Om" helps us understand our place in the universe and the universe's place within us.

These techniques are all useful to assist in becoming and staying present. Too often our thoughts linger on situations that have already passed or the mind skips ahead to daydream about the future. Meditation is the chance to be liberated from the exhausting responsibility of always being "on." This way, we're not in the past or the future—we are witnessing what is happening right now, in the present. We are not the thoughts or emotions that float in and out, we start to see ourselves in our true role as the "seer" behind those experiences.

Above all, it isn't bad to have thoughts or emotions that surface. In fact, they may serve a purpose or have a lesson to teach us. The mindset that we have in this practice is the top priority. Rather than beating ourselves up, we are given the chance to be kind, compassionate, and patient. As the seer, all that we can hope for is the willingness to "catch" ourselves in those moments when the mind wanders, then to have the strength to come back to the focus waiting for us in the present.

3

PRANAYAMA

THE ENERGY OF BREATH

Pranayama can be loosely translated to "prana" or "pran"—with multiple meanings, in this case referring to breath—and "ayam(a)", implying control or extension. Both interpretations are useful to uncover the purpose behind these practices. Control, in the sense that pranayama encourages focus—connecting the conscious mind and subconscious with breathing—while extension alludes to the unobstructed flow of breath. Breath is the foundation of any yoga practice. Becoming intentional with breath can spark drastic shifts in awareness, presence, and energetic state. Breathing happens effortlessly, yet when applied to a mindfulness practice, it transforms into a powerful tool.

The act of breathing itself really is a miracle. Here we are, having this meaningful exchange with the world—taking in air full of prana—life-force energy—trading up carbon dioxide (CO_2) for the oxygen necessary to our survival, while the CO_2 released supports the life of organic matter. This is a reminder of a symbiotic relationship that exists naturally, an act of complete perfection. This simple yet profound occurrence is an event to cultivate so much gratitude towards. It is breath that gives us life and provides us with opportunities to be more present.

The ancient yogis knew of the overwhelming potential of harnessing our breath for overall health, not to mention its potential to give rise to elevated states of consciousness. When used intentionally, breath can be a way of "checking in" by creating more awareness of what's occurring in the present. Physical sensations, thoughts, emotions, and fluctuations all become very apparent when breath is a focal point. With a keen focus, breath provides messages hidden in the unconscious mind.

I never realized how much breath mattered until I became fully aware of my breath throughout the day. When I started to "tap in" to this strength, everything changed. After this shift, I returned home from a training with a heightened awareness of my breath. I noticed fluctuations as I got back into my routine that gave me a lot of insight into what I was feeling.

One day, I entered an empty elevator by myself. On the next floor, a group of about 6 men walked in laughing and talking away—it was clear they were all close, either friends, family, or colleagues. These men seemed friendly, approachable and nothing they said was mildly intimidating, yet I could feel this sense of overwhelm wash over me.

My breath was slightly "off"—it became shorter, shallower, and less steady—my heart began to pick up the pace. I could feel the anxiety building inside of me. I had no idea before this moment that me, alone in an elevator with 6 or so regular, average Joes could provoke this kind of fear. I had been in similar situations, but I had never stopped to fully feel what was happening in my breath.

Beyond the role that breath plays in increasing awareness, the energetic connection of conscious breathing has powerful implications for healing. Unprocessed emotional patterns can be stored in the body's tissues including muscle, fascia, and even organs. By ignoring strong emotions, the body will hold onto them until they can't be overlooked any longer.

Anger, sadness, grief, and anxiety are just a few reactions that can shift from an energetic field into a physical symptom manifested as tension, pain, or disease. Experiencing a range of emotions is part of a healthy, human experience. Problems only start happening when the body chooses to hold onto intense emotions so that there's nowhere else to go, so they get "stuck."

These stuck emotions are stored in the body through cells that make up tissues. Being open to feeling, reflecting, and honouring what comes up emotionally will make it possible for these feelings to flow through without getting stuck energetically. Stepping out of this trap of pushing things down or bottling them up teaches the value of learning to let go. "Letting go" meaning the decision to stop ruminating on anything that can't be controlled.

The art of letting go can be supported by using the breath to its full potential. Creating this space is essential to your health as it will prevent disease related to stored emotions while simultaneously charging up your energetic field to radiate your light. Pranayama is the magical element that clears space for growth in both departments. Each technique holds specific intentions for your wellbeing, yet all of these offerings compliment the nervous system in deep relaxation and contribute to the radiance of the aura—the electromagnetic field around each of us.

Are all pranayama appropriate for me?

If you have a condition, please discuss with your doctor—you can even show them this book—to figure out whether a pranayama is appropriate for you. Breath holds are not suggested for those who are pregnant or have high blood pressure. With pregnancy, blood volume changes, plus, on an energetic-level it is better to have an unobstructed flow of prana for the fetus.

Breath-holding for those with high blood pressure causes further increases of blood pressure to potentially dangerous levels. For all other conditions, there are certain pranayama that are less accessible, however, there are steps that can help—including the use of a neti pot.

Get Yourself a Neti Pot!

If you've never used a neti pot before, congratulations! This bit of information is a game-changer. If you have used a neti pot before but haven't gotten the hang of it or you find yourself terrified to use it, then get ready to have your mind blown—just bear with me. For those who are new to the idea, a neti pot is a device that looks like a tea pot filled with saline solution meant for nasal irrigation.

The benefits to using a neti pot are staggering. A 2009 study showed that using a neti pot cleanses your nasal cavity—perfect for breath flow—and even removes inflammatory-causing elements that will improve your respiratory system's ability to self-clean. Clearing out the gunk in your airways can prevent colds and flus while creating space for energy to flow easefully through prana.

When I started to use a neti pot regularly, my sinuses felt amazing and even my eyes were clearer and brighter. My first experience with neti potting was well before I became a yoga teacher—I gave up almost immediately. My initial reaction was, "Ugh it feels like I'm drowning!" or "Ack, I can't get it to go through to the other side!" I had no one to "show me the ropes" so to speak so it felt like I was trying to hit a bullseye in the dark. Years later, when I finally had someone show me, with some practice, it was easy! Luckily for you, this will set the record straight so that you can be successful too.

Start by purchasing a neti pot which can be found online or in most pharmacies and health stores. These will sometimes come as a "kit" which will have the right salt supplied but, if you are acquiring only the neti pot you will also need to get iodine and preservative-free salt —NOT table salt. It's common to see specific labels stating "neti pot salt" online or at the store.

Having clean water is an extremely important step—tap water alone is not sanitized enough unless it has been boiled. Boil tap water in a kettle and let it cool. To rapidly cool the water, place a metal or stainless steel water bottle of the boiled water in the sink full of cold water, 5 – 10 minutes later it will be cool enough to put in the neti pot. Add the salt (1 – 3 tsps), then fill ½ the neti pot with the cold pre-boiled water, then top up with a few splashes of the hot boiled water. Pour out a small amount on your finger to check the temperature.

When it feels comfortably "warm" (rather than hot) then set it against the inside of one of your nostrils. The idea is that the salt water is like the constitution of the fluids in your body which will make the sensations of the water passing through the nasal cavity more comfortable.

The next "trick" is the head tilt. Your head will need to tilt forward and to the side facing towards your neti pot. For example, if the neti pot is in your right nostril, you'll need to tilt your head forward and look to your right. This "head tilt" takes a bit of practice but once you have it you can comfortably funnel the saline solution in one side so that it streams out of the other nostril. While it's streaming through, breathe in and out of your mouth. If a bit of the solution comes out of your mouth, that is also normal.

Finally, the trick to being consistent with your neti pot: leave your neti pot out next to your toothbrush—or in an obvious place—rather than stuffed in a drawer or under the sink. If it's "out" you'll remember to use it, when it's tucked away it's easy to forget about it.

Proudly display your neti pot in a spot where you'll see it consistently —to use once or even twice a day, preferably before practicing pranayama, to clear your passageways for breath and to enhance its effects. To make prepping the solution easier, cool the water the day before and leave in a water bottle in the fridge so it's ready to go.

WHEN IS IT USEFUL TO PRACTICE PRANAYAMA?

Traditionally, most pranayama is practiced first or close to the beginning of the sequence, since it assists with "dropping in" to a relaxed state through focus and prompting the flow of prana. With that said, this is not a hard rule. Checking in or using pranayama at other points in your practice, particularly as a transition or before savasana, also holds plenty of value. Use this as a suggestion to experiment! Become a yoga-scientist and get curious about how pranayama can be used to heighten presence. The following choices of pranayama are tools to add to your toolbox to make it happen.

Pranayama can be practiced anywhere from 3 – 10+ minutes—feel free to use more than one technique in your sequence.

Benefits of Pranayama

Currently, science is only scratching the surface regarding research on pranayama. Numerous scientific journals have looked at the benefits of various breathing techniques used in yoga, yet most studies have focused on the nervous system, pulmonary system, circulatory system, and stress.

One study even linked yogic breathing to a reduction in oxidative stress, associated with aging and disease. Although these studies have begun to demonstrate the power of pranayama, the ancient yogis knew there was so much more depth to these traditions.

When practiced sincerely, the subtle nature of prana promotes healing for the physical body in so many ways aside from what's happening physiologically—mostly accredited to stress relief. As practitioners, it's important to recognise that there are benefits derived from scientific research and benefits associated with traditional, yogic perspectives.

Favouring either approach does the other a disservice. Both can live harmoniously! With a traditional approach, the sages throughout history have predicted, absorbed, and intuitively downloaded information that will not be widely known for centuries to come.

Both methodologies—traditional and research-based—can be respected for their contribution to yoga as a whole. The pranayama listed in this chapter are linked to a decrease in sympathetic activity—associated with benefits from scientific research—while the additional benefits mentioned are derived from a traditional lens unless stated otherwise.

SAMA VRITTI—OR EVEN BREATHING (WITH OR WITHOUT BREATH HOLDS)

Even breathing, as the name suggests, allows for an even amount of time for each inhalation and exhalation. This is extremely useful when seeking steadiness and stability as it offers an intense focus on counting.

Avoidances

Avoid the breath holds (just inhale and exhale evenly) if you are pregnant or have high blood pressure.

How to

Inside your head, repeat the following after an exhale: Inhale – 2 – 3 – 4, Hold (your breath) – 2 – 3 – 4 Exhale – 2 – 3 – 4, Hold – 2 – 3 – 4 (repeat)

You can increase the amount of counts to 6, 8 or even 10+ as long as each section of breath is even (i.e. inhales, exhales, and holds are all the same number)

Benefits

Fosters steadiness and stability. Breath holds are useful for energetic retention and circulation. Has the potential to create powerful focus.

VISHAMA VRITTI—OR UNEVEN BREATHING (WITH OR WITHOUT BREATH HOLDS)

Uneven breathing takes the cake as one of the most grounding pranayama. If you're looking for a way to "land", vishama vritti will not only anchor you down, it'll provide you with roots.

Avoidances

None

How to

Inside your head, repeat the following after an exhale: Inhale – 2 – 3 – 4, Exhale – 2 – 3 – 4 – 5 – 6

You can increase the amount of counts to 6, 8 or even 10+ given that your exhale is at least 2 counts longer than your inhale

Benefits

Supports apana vaya, the downward and outward flow of prana. Useful for "landing" in the present—resonates strongly with qualities of the 1st chakra.

Clearing Breaths

If an emotional release is what you're after, look no further than clearing breaths. Like a sigh of relief, a clearing breath holds space for letting go of what's no longer working energetically. Clearing breaths can also be used to transition between postures.

Avoidances

None

How to

Take a deep inhale, let your exhale fall out of your mouth.

Practice 1 – 10 times

Benefits

Clearing breaths release tension in the face and jaw while creating space for emotional freedom. So much tension is held in our jaw—from anger, frustration, or holding back your thoughts—this is the chance to release that bottled up emotion.

BRAHMARI—OR BEE BREATHING

Brahmari is known as the magical pranayama. Creating healing vibrations for the brain and body, this approach provides a deep sense of calm often associated with the "yoga-high." With this heightened sense of awareness, it's easy to see why this technique feels so nourishing for the soul.

Avoidances

None

How to

Brahmari sounds like the "mmm" at the end of "Om." Take a long exhale, inhale, then hum "mmmmmm…." Repeat.

Traditionally practiced with fingertips resting on the scalp and "closing off" the ears using thumbs over the inner ear flap. However, variations of mudras* are welcomed including placing palms on various parts of your body.

*mudra translates to "seal" or "gesture" referring to a symbolic or ritual gesture. Some can be done with the entire body but most are practiced through the hands and/or fingers.

Practice 3 – 20+ rounds

Note: the traditional mudra practiced involves taking your fingers on top of your head then placing your thumb over the inner ear flap to cover your ear hole—this will block out most if not all sound. You are welcome to experiment by pairing other mudras with this pranayama as well.

Benefits

A study published by Weitzberg and Lundberg revealed that humming greatly increased nasal nitrous oxide. Nitrous Oxide is a compound found in the body that causes blood vessels to widen and is known to stimulate the release of certain hormones, including insulin—relating to blood sugar regulation—and human growth hormone—sought after for strength building, muscle growth, and recovery among other essential functions.

Based on this research, the humming of brahmari can be used to promote heart health, enhance sport performance and recovery, and support healing related to circulatory issues.

On an energetic level, brahmari has the unique benefit of activating yet relaxing different areas of the brain. It is believed to support neuroendocrine function and brain health while sharing an energetic connection with the 6th and 7th chakra. Scientific research revealed that brahmari improves cognitive function by enhancing inhibition and reaction time (Saoiji et al).

These healing vibrations can also be used to "target" specific areas to address injuries, concerns, and energetic blocks. When brahmari is used intentionally, it can create freedom for any energetic space.

DIRGHA PRANAYAMA—OR THREE PART BREATHING

Simple yet effective, dirgha pranayama will help you remember what it really means to breathe.

Avoidances

If there has been a recent internal surgery, rib fracture, hernia, or any other internal concerns, focus on making this breath soft (rather than going to the height of your inhale and depth of your exhale) and avoid forcefulness completely.

How to

If using hands, set one palm on your lower belly, the other rests over your heart (can be practiced with or without hands).

Send breath into low belly, mid belly and upper chest... all the way into collarbones. Exhaling as everything softens towards your spine. Repeat.

Benefits

Dirgha pranayama allows for awareness regarding the full potential of your breath. Beyond the benefits of recognizing breath capacity, this technique offers freedom for the belly—a place that often holds so much tension.

Societal expectations contribute to plenty of shame in this area—implying that unless your belly is perfectly flat and sculpted, it is not worthy of being "liked." This garbage belief needs to be thrown out the window so we can reclaim our power.

Even the thinnest, fittest people will have space in their belly when they are taking a full inhale! Don't feel afraid to take up space in order to release the tension associated with shame and guilt. Let breath flow into your belly with radical acceptance.

SITALI/SITAKARI (ALSO KNOWN AS SHEETALI/SHEETAKARI OR "COOLING BREATHS")

If you ever find yourself with a "hot head", sitali and sitakari are the remedy. Like jumping into a cool lake on a hot summer's day, this technique is known to bring the temperature down on excess heat—physically, emotionally, and spiritually.

. . .

Avoidances

None

How to

Sitali: Start with an exhale, then stick your tongue out of your mouth. Curl it to create a straw. Inhale through the straw, exhale out of your nose (mouth closed). Repeat.

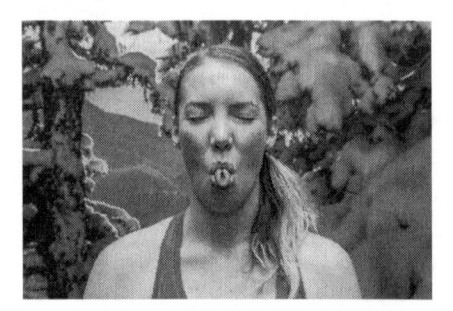

Fig. 3.2

About 30% of the population is genetically unable to curl their tongue** if you fall into that category, practice sitakari instead: Start with an exhale, then stick your tongue out of your mouth, take your tongue lightly between your teeth. Inhale through the sides of your mouth (with teeth on tongue), close your mouth to exhale through nose. Repeat.

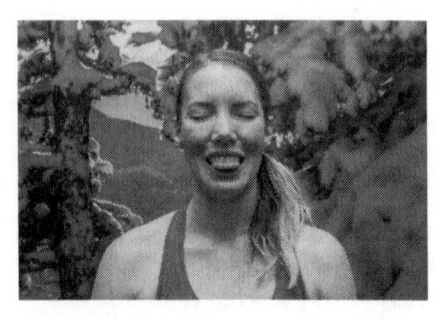

Fig. 3.3

How long

Practice sitali or sitakari for 3 – 10 minutes.

Benefits

Anger and frustration are emotions that tend to crank up the heat. Chinese medicine states that the liver is inclined to hold onto heat that stems from intense emotions. This breath technique offers the chance to put those fires out. The ancient yogis also believed this practice supported the body in detoxifying—with its cooling effects, it's clear there may be physical and energetic connections to this claim. At first the breath can taste quite bitter, but with time it may get sweeter, which is thought to be from the detoxification process.

UJAYYI BREATHING—OR "OCEANS BREATH" ALSO KNOWN AS "VICTORIOUS BREATH"

Typically used in vinyasa or hatha practices, ujayyi offers some unique benefits in restorative yoga. Connecting to the energy of the throat, ujayyi has an audible sound, making it a straightforward pranayama to cultivate focus. It is also the only technique recommended for restorative that produces heat or "tapas." Tapas is known as the light or fire that burns up impurities physically and energetically, making ujayyi the only truly relaxing pranayama that fits this intention.

Avoidances

None

How to

If ujayyi is new to you, start by taking a hand in front of your face. Inhale through your nose, exhale out of your mouth as if you're fogging a mirror. Do that two more times. Then, close your lips. Breathe with that same intention of fogging a mirror (keeping lips closed). Bring that constriction at the back of your throat to each inhalation and exhalation. This constriction in the back of your throat is known as jalandar bandha, or neck lock, with your chin ever so slightly tucked. Maintain jalandar bandha for inhalations and exhalations to bring an ocean-like audible quality to your breath.

How long

3 – 10+ minutes.

Benefits

Clearer communication and connection to truth are charged up thanks to the contribution from the 5th chakra. Ujayyi will also serve you well if you seek clarity on any given situation. When we clear space in the throat, we make way for our thoughts to work harmoniously with our speech so that we can share what's in our heart.

NADI SHODHANA—OR ALTERNATE NOSTRIL BREATHING

Nadi Shodhana is a technique that's meant to encourage balance, physically and energetically. The fascinating part about this pranayama is that it can be energizing or uplifting, depending on what needs balancing. There are many different techniques and variations of nadi shodhana; the how-to below it just one way to practice this pranayama.

Avoidances

Any sinus issues that block off one or both nasal passages.

How to

Fold the first two fingers of your right hand into you palm.

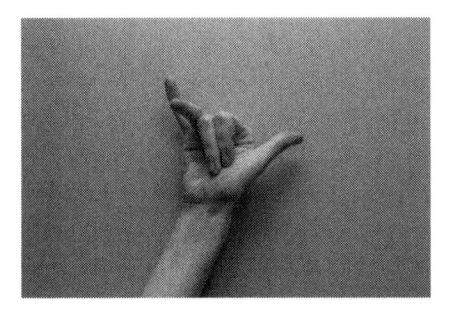

Fig. 2.4

Set your thumb on the outside of your right nostril and gently press on the outside of your nose to close off your nostril. Exhale through your left nostril. Inhale through your left nostril. Use your ring finger to close off the left nostril and release thumb from your right nostril to exhale through your right nostril. Inhale through your right nostril —close—exhale through your left nostril. Continue at your own pace for 3 – 10+ minutes. For simplicity, the "change over" always happens at the top of your inhale.

Benefits

The coordination required to practice nadi shodhana with ease can confront the two hemispheres of the brain, similarly to how difficult it can be to rub your head and pat your belly at the same time. This movement and coordination is thought to challenge different areas of the brain simultaneously.

On an energetic level, nadi shodhana invites balance between two perceived opposites known as "Ida" and "Pingala." These are known as the nadis or energetic channels. The Hatha Yoga Pradipika asserts that over 72,000 nadis run through us to support the subtle body—our energetic field fueled by prana or life force—Ida and Pingala just happen to be two out of the three that are seen as the most influential. Ida is regarded as the lunar, cooling, nurturing, energy that draws strength from the divine feminine whereas Pingala is the hot, intense, masculine energy that resonates with the sun. Ida and Pingala dance back and forth over the Sushumna—or the central channel—crossing at each chakra. They originate in Muladhara, the 1st chakra, and meet again at Ajna, the 6th chakra.

When the two are brought into balance from energetic practices—like nadi shodhana—they draw closer towards the Sushumna or central channel. The Sushumna creates a beautiful flow between the root chakra and the crown, when this is open and flowing easefully we can live joyously. If the three primary nadis are harmonious, the journey to our highest self—the one that knows true peace—is much clearer.

Final Notes For All Pranayama

Pranayama creates space for prana to flow freely. This can be a useful tactic for "dropping in" just as meditation is the path to exploring the inner landscape. Pranayama and meditation are often used interchangeably, especially because practicing pranayama can be very meditative. Think of pranayama as a potential "key" to the gate that leads down the same path as meditation. Once that gate is opened, there are effective methods of staying on this path, with meditation techniques to remain in this state of bliss.

4

RESTORATIVE PROPS

WHAT KIND, WHAT SIZE, AND HOW MANY?

The general rule in restorative yoga regarding props is "the more the merrier." To practice this style of yoga with grace and ease, the value of having adequate support cannot be understated. Although not all postures require every single prop, having them available will make the transitions between postures much easier. Unnecessary searching or confusion is avoided when these tools are ready to use. These considerations will reduce the need for alertness during the sequence —or series of postures—which means the nervous system can remain in a state of relaxation.

"What kind, what size, and how many" are common questions with regards to props. The answer: it depends. The additional factors you ought to consider are the postures you'd like to practice and whether you are healing from a specific injury that requires more attention.

In cases of injury or certain sensitivities, access to additional props is essential. Even for students who don't have injuries or concerns, using support is a requirement, whether it's the use of specific yoga props or less conventional tools.

Typical props for restorative yoga include a yoga mat, bolsters, blocks, blankets, straps, sandbags, and eye pillows while the less conventional options include items you could easily find at home—couch cushions, pillows, couches, and walls. The key to applying this gear is to use enough support that allows for complete relaxation into the posture without holding, struggling, or any form of discomfort.

Bolsters

Having a bolster available makes many postures accessible thanks to their large size and the additional support they provide. These advantages make this prop a foundational tool in this style of yoga. Pillows don't quite cut it in comparison due to their unique shape. Bolsters are generally used to support underneath major body parts—torso, back, or hips for example—but serve other purposes as well, including being a comfortable seat to sit on for meditation.

There are different sizes for bolsters, each with a specific objective. Acquiring a larger bolster while using a blanket in place of a smaller bolster can be a great option especially if space is an issue for a home practice. There are round and rectangular bolsters—the choice is based on preference. Round bolsters generally transfer more easily to a wider variety of shapes. Examples of using bolsters:

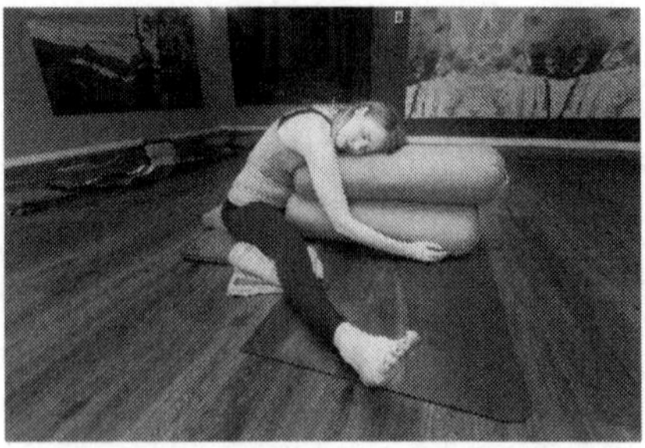

Fig. 4.1 Bolsters placed underneath to support chest and head

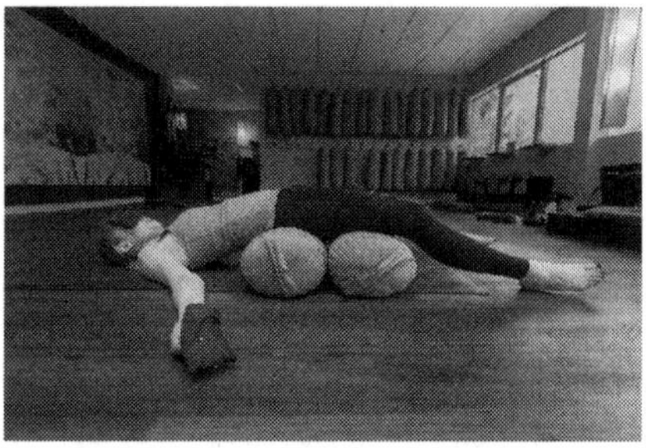

Fig. 4.2 Bolsters under hips and legs

Blocks

Blocks tend to be rectangular in shape and have varying levels of thickness. Typically they are made from wood, cork, or foam. Each shape and material holds its own benefits. For instance, a foam chip block is much thinner and wider, making it the perfect amount of lift to sit on.

Larger cork blocks on the other hand can create firmer support for lifting bolsters and blankets. Softer foam tends to be better if you are using it directly on your body, for example, when it rests underneath your forehead in a supported sphinx.

Cork blocks are more effective when they are needed for steadiness and stability with more height, as in a forward fold when set underneath bolsters. A blanket can be laid on top of a cork block to make it softer and more versatile.

Blocks can be used to provide additional lift for bolsters, as depicted below, or to support underneath knees or thighs. Examples of using blocks:

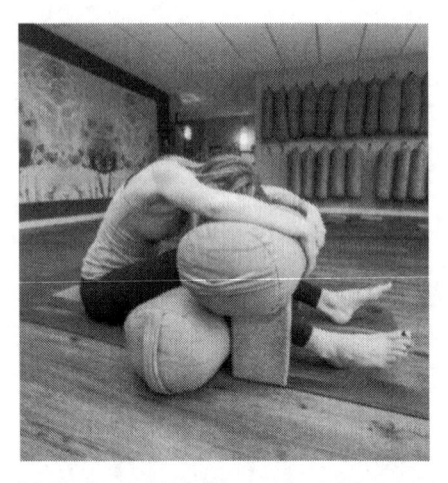

Fig. 4.3 Blocks used to further prop up bolsters to create adequate support for the upper body

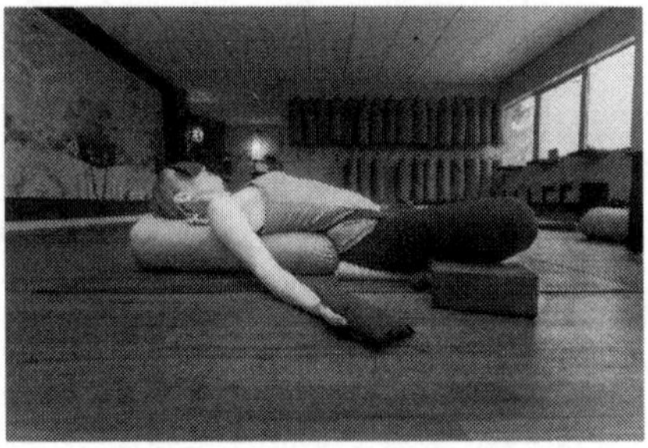

Fig. 4.4 Blocks underneath knees/thighs

Straps

Deterring leg movement is one significant benefit of using a strap. This would be useful to prevent legs from splaying out wide in legs up the wall, seated forward folds or even twists.

A strap can also create additional support and comfort for the lower back in shapes such as supta baddha konasana over a bolster, aka reclined butterfly pose (over a bolster). When the loop around the lower back is done correctly in this posture, it places gentle pressure around the sacrum and lower lumbar vertebrae which decompresses the spine.

Ultimately, it is meant to create more space for the lower back which can be very helpful for those with lower back issues or anyone who feels they need more freedom in their lower back. Examples of using straps:

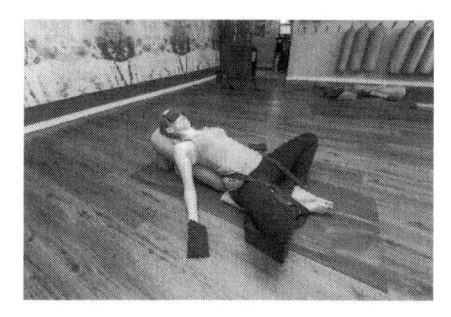

Fig. 4.5 Creating more support for the hips and decompressing the lower back

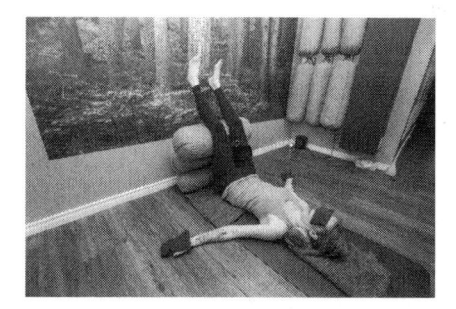

Fig. 4.6 Strap around the legs to keep them steady and stable (rather than falling open)

Blankets

The versatility of blankets makes them an essential tool for a restorative practice, at home or in the studio. They are easy to fold, roll, and manipulate into the exact shape that you need support for, or simply to provide comfort with warmth. Since restorative yoga encourages students to stay comfortable in postures for a long period of time, body temperature can be a concern.

Even a room that seems warm upon entry might start to feel chilly by the end of the practice. Making sure the temperature is comfortable will support the nervous system in relaxing, therefore making blankets a key ingredient to have close to your mat.

Blankets are also wonderful when placed between "hovering spaces" including legs in reclined twists, between hips and heels in child's pose, or to support under your neck when lying down. Examples of using blankets:

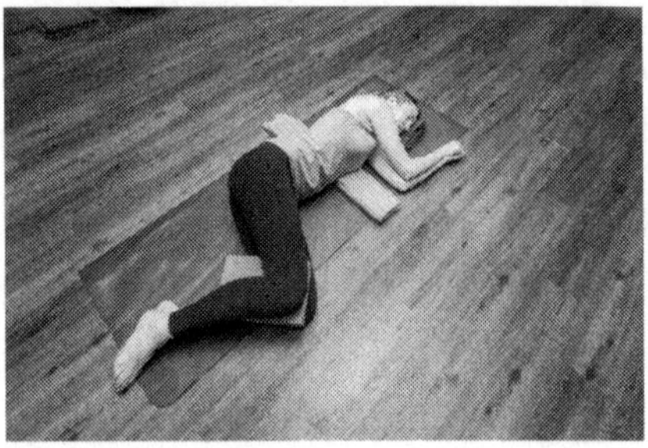

Fig. 4.7 Blanket under the largest part of the ribs to change the shape of the body, thereby creating a gentle side opening

Sandbags

Sandbags are typically 5 – 15 lbs bags that are used therapeutically by applying weight to solid structures of the body. In terms of their therapeutic qualities, they have similar effects emotionally and psychologically to weighted blankets.

"Weighted blankets have been around for a long time, especially for kids with autism or behavioral disturbances," says Dr. Cristina Cusin, an assistant professor of psychiatry at Harvard Medical School. "It is one of the sensory tools commonly used in psychiatric units.

Patients who are in distress may choose different types of sensory activities — holding a cold object, smelling particular aromas, manipulating dough, building objects, doing arts and crafts — to try to calm down."

Another study by Hayduke and Nye looked at the effect of weighted blankets on children who are on the autism spectrum. Their results showed a correlation between weighted blanket use with improved quality and quantity of sleep. Sandbags, like weighted blankets, give additional weight in certain postures to deliver a relaxing sensory experience for students. It is important that sandbags are used only on solid structures—bones for example—so that it does not impede breathing, organs, or soft tissue. Sandbags are perfect to use on legs, shoulders, arms, pelvis or feet in supported postures.

An important note for women: do not use sandbag across the front of the pelvis (laid across both hip bones) during pregnancy. It is also not recommended during menstruation. Example of using sandbags:

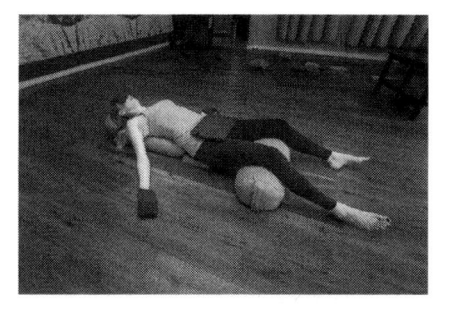

Fig. 4.8 Across the hips

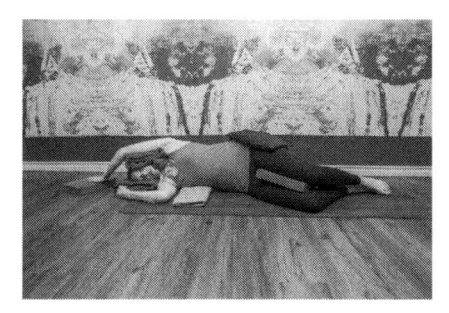

Fig. 4.9 On the side of the hip

Eye Pillows

Eye pillows are one of my all-time favourite props. They parallel the benefits of sandbags in the sense that they also provide additional weight which is very therapeutic, even though they are significantly lighter. When used over the eyes they also block out any light, allowing for deeper relaxation. The pineal gland located in the brain is very sensitive to light and is responsible for the production of melatonin. A study from Gooley et al. suggested that exposure to room light before bedtime suppresses melatonin onset and production duration.

Melatonin is the hormone responsible for sleep regulation and circadian rhythm. If the focus of a restorative practice is to sleep better, this is important knowledge to integrate. For those practicing before bed, it would be a considerable advantage to practice using an eye pillow. Although more research is required, I do feel that eye pillows are beneficial for the health of the pineal gland at any point in time. With regular exposure to artificial, harsh indoor light, to experience complete darkness in addition to weight is a gift to the nervous system.

Spiritually, it also connects us to one of the 8 limbs of yoga known as pratyhara, or sense withdrawal. This value asks us to take a step back from constant stimulation, particularly through our eyes and ears, granting us the ability to better understand our inner landscape. Figure 4.8 above is an excellent example of using eye pillows over eyes and in hands. Non-traditional props can include items that you already have in your home. Blankets, couch pillows, eye masks, folded pillow cases or sheets can all be substituted as yoga props under the right circumstances. Use them freely in your restorative practice as long as enough of them are supplied with adequate shape to create support.

5

INJURIES, ILLNESS, AND RADICAL TRANSFORMATION

I broke my wrist one winter, an injury that required surgery to screw a plate into one of the bones in my forearm. This experience came with plenty of lessons. It was difficult in the physical sense since my arm was immobile for some time, but there were also a rollercoaster of emotions to cope with. I had challenges with basic day-to-day tasks that became frustrating and emotionally draining. My yoga practice which normally gave me comfort and consistency had become clunky and inaccessible.

I had to change the way that I looked at asana, even the basic postures I'd practiced for many years. This included a "no-arm" sun salutation along with a modified restorative practice. On my healing journey it became clear that being injured added another layer of spiritual training. Throughout this path I would have to redefine what "yoga" was, what it looked like, and develop radical honesty—I knew that the courage to choose conscious relaxation would coax my nervous system to reinforce the healing process. Despite the challenges I faced, my practice supported me in ways I hadn't anticipated. It gave me the confidence to know that yoga would always be there for me, even when certain postures were off the table.

Shortly after this experience, I met a woman by the name of Mary-Jo Fetterly, a restorative yoga practitioner and yoga teacher who is a quadriplegic. She teaches adaptive yoga for those with physical and cognitive disabilities. To see her overcome the barriers associated with mobility to create a truly inclusive practice was inspiring. After seeing this first-hand, I understood that anyone could adapt a yoga practice with the right tools, knowledge, and conviction.

Mindset can be a struggle for those with injuries, illness, or other limitations. Specifically, when it comes to adopting their own practice and choosing the appropriate modifications. This is one of the greatest challenges a student will face as a yoga practitioner. Honesty, bravery, and strength are fundamental to honouring one's unique set of circumstances—a standard that must be followed with any form of yoga.

This means that your choices reflect the needs of your body, mind, and spirit regardless of the choices other students make, or the expectations that are imposed on you by yourself or your teacher. Often, when there is a hesitancy to change, it comes from a place of fear related to shame and judgement. Most students will settle with being uncomfortable rather than "going against the grain."

The thought of doing something different than their teacher or peers triggers feelings of worthlessness or rejection. Following directions is a basic tenet developed during childhood. Recognizing the harmful potential of this outlook is necessary to release these patterns—which are useful in some cases—but we must learn where these rules are meant to be broken. In restorative yoga, these are the moments to become empowered, by choosing physical comfort, even if it means creating temporary mental or emotional discomfort in doing so. There are a few warning signs to look out for when honouring the practice of restorative yoga.

PAIN OR DISCOMFORT

Medical News Today defines pain as an unpleasant sensation and emotional experience linked to tissue damage. The body is meant to react with signals in order to prevent any further harm. Discomfort on the other hand may not be sharpness or "pain", but any sensation that draws your attention to that area which takes you out of your present experience. This can be subtle, meaning that practicing with mindfulness, care, and honesty is required to find the opportunities to invite relaxation instead of suffering.

TINGLING OR NUMBNESS

Sensations of tingling or numbness indicate pressure or restriction on a nerve. This can happen in a variety of restorative postures. For instance, when practicing a reclined twist, the brachial plexus—a cluster of nerves along the anterior (front) surface of the shoulder—can experience compression when the arm is outstretched.

The simplest way to alleviate the pressure is to shift out of the shape completely. In the reclined twist example, rolling all the way over to one side can alleviate the discomfort relatively quickly. Once you've returned to a comfortable state, then practice the shape with additional support. In this case it's a good idea to use a blanket to prop yourself up either under your shoulder or knees to reduce the intensity of the release.

STRETCHING

Switching your thinking from "doing" to doing less is a perspective to embrace in order to receive many of the benefits restorative yoga offers. Many students crave sensation, whether it's strength derived from active yoga postures or the feeling of stretching from shapes that are more passive and static. Restorative yoga asks us to do neither, by avoiding strong sensations altogether, thereby embracing the transformation that comes from doing less.

To practice restorative yoga effectively, the difference between stretching and releasing must be understood. A stretch is a strong sensation that creates mild to strong discomfort whereas the process involved in a release is experienced as an unwinding of tension—one that is subtle and blissful.

UNCONSCIOUS HOLDING

Holding onto unnecessary tension and tightness is a common response to stress. Even when the body is finally given the chance to fully relax, these reactions tend to hang around. Awareness is the antidote for the lingering symptoms in response to stressful events. Practicing a full body scan, from your toes out all the way up to your head, can be useful in uncovering what areas are triggered by stress.

Feet

- Toes tend to scrunch—invite them to soften instead
- Arches can hold tension—allow feet to relax

Legs

- Contraction often held in thighs, either quadriceps or hamstrings—let your legs get heavy

Pelvis

- Gluteals tend to hold a contraction, along with the psoas (a major hip flexor) on the front of the pelvis—relax the areas around your pelvis

Back

- Erector spinae, a set of muscles along the spine, tend to maintain tension—soften the muscles that support your spine

Note: you will still maintain the natural curvature of your spine, which will change shape based on the posture you practice

Shoulders

- Commonly shrug up towards ears or slouch forward—let them relax with the weight of gravity according to the posture.

Neck

- Front and back of the neck can be tense from stress which can result in tension along the back of the head or the scalp as well—keep the back of your neck long, soften the muscles around your throat

Face and Head

- Muscles of the face tend to scrunch. Especially the jaw, forehead, and between the brows—invite all of these areas to soften instead

- Let the back of your head get heavier

Certain postures can trigger patterns of unconscious holding. Intention is everything when it comes to finding relaxation. For example, relaxing your shoulders will look and feel different in a forward fold vs. a heart opener.

In a forward fold shoulders will naturally roll forward with gravity—an action known as protraction. Shoulders in a reclined heart opener however will slightly retract, an action when the scapulas—or shoulder blades on the back of your body—move closer towards each other. In these two circumstances the intention is quite different since completing the same action—either protraction or retraction—will result in relaxation for one posture and tension in the other. Understanding intention is an essential step in revealing how to relax in each shape. The body will naturally tell you which direction feels "right" as gravity will assist in the relaxation process.

TAPAS, TECHNOLOGY, AND DISTRACTIONS

"Tapas" is an observance followed by those who walk the path of yoga, often referring to tenacity or discipline. This notion holds many translations including "austerity" or "to heat" but also refers to the ability "to burn" or "to change." Regardless of the interpretation of tapas, this lesson should be at the forefront of any yoga practice. Without the purpose sparked by tapas, there is no drive to set foot on your mat everyday. Without the heat or light within ourselves energetically, there is no passion, fire, or spark, which breeds dullness.

Tapas is the internal drive that lights the fire under our ass that we all need to accomplish our goals. The home of the fire that lives within each of us rests in the 3rd chakra, manipura—a place with the potential to burn up impurities physically or spiritually. The lower chakras are associated with survival and therefore tend to hold onto fear. When we shift our energy upwards, it passes through the fire of the 3rd chakra before it enters the heart, the gatekeeper of the higher chakras.

These higher energy centers are related to the qualities that resonate with our highest potential, including love, truth, and connection. These states, thoughts, and actions have a higher vibrational frequency than their negative counterparts— fear, judgement, and apathy. Every choice we make has a vibrational frequency. Having an awareness of the energetic consequences of our thoughts and actions gives us the power to choose how our spiritual anatomy evolves.

That doesn't mean that every moment is perfect, having these reactions is normal—we are human beings who are meant to be flawed—the key is to use tapas to "catch" ourselves in those moments, thereby consciously choosing to connect with the virtues that align with our highest self.

Tapas also makes an appearance in the conditions that surround our yoga practice, particularly in regard to technology. Having the discipline to step away from your phone or other devices is part of your commitment when you set foot on the mat. I've heard many excuses over the years but there are very few legitimate reasons to stay "on" constantly. Even with a packed schedule, stepping away for one hour is possible.

The idea that it is a requirement to be "on" and "available" relentlessly reflects a sickness of the mind resulting in a physical manifestation of disease if it goes unaddressed. Often this thinking comes from the need to always be "doing" since success is associated with achievement. This misguided belief must be reframed in order to heal. For the individuals that cope with stress, intensity, and pressure on a regular basis, stillness will always be medicine. That stillness is born out of the discipline (tapas) to understand that relaxation is a necessity rather than luxury.

Other distractions can be a barrier for some students, especially when practicing at home. Even if you practice regularly at a studio, developing a home practicing is an asset. Practicing in a home environment may be convenient but it shares its own unique challenges. Having access to personal comforts and entertainment can be a diversion while students who cohabit or live in noisy neighborhoods face additional hurdles.

Understanding how to practice under these conditions is a blessing. After all, if we wait for everything to be "perfect"—perfect lighting, perfect quiet, perfect ambiance—the time will never come. I have even experienced this in yoga studios with the most beautiful, blissful ambiance. Construction, an event, or an overly enthusiastic pedestrian all have one thing in common: they all have the potential to remove bliss. However, it is a choice whether those circumstances make an impact.

We must embrace the imperfections that are brought as gifts. These "distractions" are obstacles that are meant to be overcome with presence through mindfulness and meditation. In these situations, these moments can be thought of as "spiritual tests" to see if the tools have been developed to cultivate presence even under pressure. We are never given any spiritual test that we aren't prepared for which means it has been presented so that we can rise to the challenge.

TIPS FOR PRACTICING AT HOME

- Either turn your phone off completely OR set it to Airplane Mode with the WiFi turned off.
- Let those you live with know not to distract you during your practice time—even if you are practicing in a shared space like a living room. Set clear boundaries.
- Embrace distractions that you can't control like pets, outside noise, or otherwise. You can give the option for children to practice with you or go somewhere else. Having a sense of humour is key in these instances.
- Those with busy schedules, commitments, and people that depend on them… let those people know you'll be "stepping out" for an hour. That may mean an e-mail alert gets activated or an automatic reply.
- Set a time and stick to it: one that makes sense for you and your schedule. Treat it with as much respect as you would for your work, appointments, and all other commitments.

Building tapas to sustain your practice demands radical honesty. Being honest involves reflecting on the triggers that prevent you from relaxation and clarity. Exercising strong boundaries for the factors you can influence is necessary, paired with the tenacity to let go of what you can't control. Surrender in this context is the only way to maintain joy.

There's no room to take ourselves too seriously, on or off the mat, so mitigate the factors you can control and embrace what you cannot. The universe likes to leave little "spiritual tests", so meet them with bravery, honesty, and a sense of humour.

6

NOT BEING A SPIRITUAL ASSHOLE

No one ever set out with the intention of being a spiritual asshole. In fact, most who are guilty of abusing the power of spirituality truly believe that they are doing the right thing. The term "spiritual asshole" applies to anyone using divine knowledge in order to belittle someone else, whether they realize it or not.

Shedding the light of awareness on this subject is the swiftest way to avoid its pitfalls. When developing an understanding of the chakras, it is clear that this philosophy holds intrinsic value, especially when it comes to personal growth. Becoming empowered with this information demands a great deal of responsibility.

It is our duty as spiritual seekers to apply these lessons in day-to-day life, thereby embodying the teachings even when the message creates discomfort or reveals unforeseen hurdles. These hurdles remind us that perfection is impossible; each teaching directs us to strive towards the best version of ourselves. Maya Angelou once said, "Do the best you can until you know better. Then when you know better, do better."

Being a spiritual asshole is easy to fall victim to, even with the best of intentions. We can do all the inner work, meditation, accumulate crystals, read tarot, and chant mantra as much as we want—but at the end of the day, we are still human. Each of us has innate needs and fears paired with a unique history and outlook on life. It's a miracle we can all communicate with each other at all! When one human being relates to another, how can we know what is helpful and what is harmful?

Although we cannot change anyone's perspective, when these concepts are articulated consciously it impacts how they are received and integrated. When the lessons of spirituality are shared freely, there is the potential to open doors or to close them.

When diving down the spiritual rabbit hole, it can be tempting to compare our stage of development to soothe the ego. Surely, after all the hard work, there must be a higher spot to take within the spiritual hierarchy? Yet it is this very thought pattern that plagues the soul's development. According to Buddhism, desire and ignorance are the root of suffering.

Comparison is a deadly form of desire destined to cause disappointment, making it easier to slip into patterns associated with being a spiritual asshole. Energetic well-being depends on us catching ourselves in those moments of comparison. A sneaky type of comparison is the "spiritual pedestal" complex that plagues earnest practitioners looking to identify with their love for spirituality.

The idea of being placed on a pedestal to flaunt spiritual awakening is one of the greatest traps on the spiritual path. Accepting the thought "I am more spiritual than you" has a toxic impact, whether it's a belief expressed inwardly or outwardly. Believing in this manifesto is a downfall that feeds the ego, leading to a separation from our higher self which has no need to equate itself with a "greater than" or "lesser than" mentality.

Someone truly spiritually evolved has no need for comparison. It is essential to recognize that we are all on a journey, whether one is fully aware of this fact or not. This path is not a "race" and there is no finish line or prize at the end. When the needs of the spirit are met, it's not necessary to prove its place in the world as superior. A competitive streak can completely hinder someone from experiencing what emerges with relaxation and subtle energetic work. Can you imagine a spiritually enlightened master seeking approval for being the most spiritual? Let this notion be a reminder that there is no "end game" or trophy when we reach an important milestone in our personal development.

Although an awakening may result in increased awareness the real value is often felt through how deeply we are able to let go by releasing lingering anger, frustration, hate, indifference, and other negative emotions—resulting in freedom for the spiritual self. We don't even have to know "how" to let go if we are willing and open for the universe to support the process. Like a winding road, sometimes the process is two steps forward and one step back which reinforces the idea of a "spiritual pedestal" as damaging to the many lessons the universe provides us with.

Realizing there's no finish line also prompts us to take judgment out of the equation when we pursue our higher self, especially with how we view other people. They too are navigating the world as best they can—some have very few skills to draw from to keep them grounded, nourished, and feeling whole. A dear reiki client of mine once confessed to me that she did not relate to her loved ones since they did not share her commitment to spirituality. This made her feel lonely and disconnected.

My response was that she should continue shining her light brightly in their presence. When we are a shining example of the lessons we absorb, those around us will naturally reflect that contagious energy. A few of my favourite people don't completely resonate with my belief system yet I notice how their perspectives have shifted over time.

Their openness echoes the work I have done on myself over the years, evidence that when we continue to "show up" energetically it generates a ripple effect. Seeing and feeling these effects through our loved ones can take time. For me, it was over many years. Having loved ones who share a similar belief structure is something to be cherished however, all relationships built on mutual respect are a treasure.

Never feel that you must give up a relationship due to a weak spiritual bond when your beliefs are appreciated and respected. If we set a good example for other people that energy will be contagious, regardless of their current belief system.

The biggest culprits when it comes to being a spiritual asshole are those who shame others for what they lack in regards to energetic health. Choosing to "diagnose" using a lecture on how to heal a chakra system is a classic move of a spiritual asshole—when this is done without being prompted for guidance it can be detrimental. The actions of this presumed spiritual savior will ultimately do more harm than good. Often these individuals have good intentions beneath their behavior but their delivery is far from helpful to the person undergoing hardship or overcoming their own demons.

Using our knowledge to empower others, rather than belittle them, is part of our responsibility as a spiritual seeker. Approaching someone with demands to improve their health energetically is the quickest way to repel them from taking the spiritual path to healing. Rather, this is an opportunity for us to hold space for them while setting healthy boundaries with them for our personal well-being. It may also be appropriate to suggest practitioners that can act as a guide on their journey—a good energetic practitioner, holistic healer, or osteopath can go a long way. No one should feel alone during the healing process, we all need a helping hand sometimes. Even with the best recommendations and the will to hold space for those we care about, we cannot control someone else's path. It is challenging to watch someone make questionable decisions, yet it is not always our place to step in as their savior.

Having to learn first hand is the only way some individuals will truly absorb their lessons to make serious changes in their life. For those who are open to seeking support, finding the right guidance is extremely valuable given the teacher or practitioner has pure intentions. There are many warm, kind-hearted, genuine souls out there to learn from however we must be aware that not all mentors have our best interests at heart.

Lording power over someone energetically creates a dangerously toxic relationship. Someone once shared this announcement, "I am your guru, I will always be your guru" to their students before leading a training. This statement is deeply concerning since a teacher is a guide, not someone to be placed on a pedestal. Whenever a mentor is put up on a pedestal it changes the student-teacher relationship by creating an environment for an unhealthy co-dependency. A corrupt student-teacher bond consists of a teacher, healer, shaman, or other holistic health practitioner who preys upon vulnerabilities that foster a dysfunctional energetic dynamic.

The vulnerable person may be made to feel that they are never "healed" or that they are always in need of more treatments, another retreat, or a specific training in order to truly be whole—they may also be manipulated with spiritual lessons to maintain this dynamic. Implanting these toxic thoughts into an impressionable mind is a common "move" for this type of spiritual asshole—caring more about their own needs while disregarding what is best for the student. Abusing this power dynamic can have numerous intended outcomes including gaining attention, adoration, greed, or sexual gratification—whatever keeps them from falling off the pedestal to ensure their needs stay met. Fortunately, it is completely possible to be open to receiving guidance without being taken advantage of.

Maintaining energetic balance in a relationship means that there is a fair exchange of energetic resources. These energetic resources can materialize as time, money, skills, knowledge, or other valuable resources. When both the teacher and student maintain healthy boundaries and respect one another for their contribution to the relationship a positive dynamic can blossom. When there is balance, respect, and sincerity between student and teacher then retreats, trainings, workshops, and classes are all wonderful ways of expanding the tools that nurture knowledge, strength, joy, understanding, and fulfillment. Preserving the condition of the relationship demands respectful boundaries on either side.

When enforcing these boundaries our responsibility is to respond with kindness and compassion—even if that means bringing up something that's hard to swallow. An incorrect perception about kindness and compassion is the idea that those who exercise these qualities are "pushovers." This perception couldn't be further from the truth. The strongest souls apply fair and clear boundaries regularly and in abundance. Often, kindness and compassion are confused with "niceness." Niceness in this context is a false narrative used to suppress emotion towards personal boundaries. Setting clear boundaries is always a kind and compassionate act.

There is one category of spiritual asshole who manipulates the tenets of yoga and spirituality to disrespect boundaries and cast judgement on others. This individual lacks the self-awareness to take responsibility for their actions—they will seek to displace blame in order to keep playing the victim. Coming across this spiritual asshole is not uncommon amongst the spiritual community. Take a yoga studio for example; it requires being clear about the rules that support everyone using the space, including all students, teachers, and staff.

The policies are in place so that everyone can thrive—following these guidelines makes it possible for operations to run smoothly. For example, at our studio we cap our classes to reduce class size, offering a unique personal experience for our students. As a practitioner, it is a major benefit to connect with your teacher while receiving quality instruction and support throughout the practice. Reinforcing this intention requires a cancellation policy which we state clearly on our website, through our online booking page, and in emailed receipts—

this allows students on the wait-list a fair opportunity to get into class. In the past, I have had the rare student who becomes frustrated when we stand our ground regarding cancellations.

I remember one email made in anger accused us of being "un-yogic" for reinforcing our rules when in fact, the opposite was true—if we let our policy slide, it would be unfair to the dedicated students who honoured their reservation. Completely disregarding something like a cancellation policy with no remorse falls under the category of a "regular asshole" but what makes a spiritual asshole is the manipulation of spiritual teachings.

When the late canceller starts to throw around terms like "unyogic" or "unkind"—in response to firm and clear boundaries—that's when these teachings are warped into something manipulative. Throwing around these accusations without personal reflection is an attempt to displace the blame and guilt. Twisting the philosophies of yoga—like kindness and compassion—is a common ploy of the spiritual asshole for the purpose of emotional manipulation. In situations like this, we can empathize with someone without being a pushover.

In fact, to act with clarity, compassion, and kindness by setting boundaries will likely save many headaches in the future. Your self-worth deserves attention, making these boundaries worthwhile even if that means bearing through childlike temper tantrums from full-grown adults. Boundaries may also include creating physical or communicative space between you and the other person for your mental and emotional health.

The final classification of the spiritual asshole is the one who divides everything into "spiritual" or "non-spiritual." Classifying types of activities, personal choices, or people as strictly one category or the other is a misguided belief. We are all spirit inhabiting a human form for our time on earth with the lessons of spirituality guiding us. Spirit touches us in its own unique way.

Some may feel the spark of their inner light while dancing to jazz while others experience that brightness listening to their favorite DJ. It is not our place to judge how others connect to their spirit. Each of us has the responsibility of being honest with ourselves about what brightens our light and what dims it. This might seem challenging at first to navigate but it's quite simple. For example, certain junk food might seem like it brings happiness in the moment but lethargy or a negative mood sets in after consuming it.

This choice would be an example of dimming your light rather than contributing to the brightness you deserve. In addition, our choices may impact the other beings that share this earth. As practitioners of yoga it is our responsibility to consider whether our actions inflict pain or suffering on others, then consciously choose the best route to be an uplifting force in the world. This can be confusing to those who naturally lean into toxic forms of kindness that always put other people's needs first. Like the old saying goes, we cannot pour from an empty cup meaning that to support ourselves on this spiritual path, our needs must be the top priority.

When uncomfortable situations arise, like telling a person something uncomfortable they need to hear, choosing a course of action is hard for anyone who does not want to inflict mental or emotional discomfort. The thought of making someone uncomfortable or upset may seem like the move of a spiritual asshole but in this context, it's quite the opposite—we are meant to stand up for ourselves lovingly. So how do we figure out what's cruel and what's kind? Using careful discernment will uncover the true meaning of compassion so that the decision becomes clear.

A close friend of mine was going through a very rough patch in her life. Substantial blows to her health had impacted every aspect of her existence. She underwent surgery after surgery and developed a serious disability within a year forcing her to cope with many major changes. We kept in touch over the phone as we lived long distance from one another.

What I noticed through this transition is that she became increasingly down and depressed with her circumstances, which was easy to empathize with. I was completely open to being a listening ear for her and had been for a long time, but I found that our phone calls became increasingly draining.

Emotionally and spiritually I felt depleted, like my entire energetic battery had been run dry following each conversation. With no sign of good news and the calls increasingly becoming one-sided it became harder and harder to pick up the phone. I felt as though I was being emotionally dumped on. Soon after, I hopped on a plane to visit her. I knew that as difficult as this conversation would be, I had to make it clear that I was no longer available for emotional dumping.

Although I would always be there for her and I wanted to support her, I had limits too. The conversation was hard. She was very upset. As challenging as it was, I felt that the weight of the situation was lifted almost instantly. After that initial band aid had been ripped off, I could feel our relationship mending.

Some readers might process that narrative and jump to believe "but, I thought we weren't supposed to be a pushover?" Let me make this clear: yes, we want to set boundaries, yet we can also give ourselves the space to forgive and continue these relationships when the person is willing to respect those boundaries going forward. Forgiveness is not a weakness. In fact, it might just be the most advanced act we can practice as spiritual seekers. And what about those who don't respect those boundaries? Luckily, forgiveness can be long-distance even if you cut ties in a relationship.

When we stand up for ourselves in these situations the feelings and actions of others cannot be controlled, even when we have the best of intentions. Taking a stand does not make you a spiritual asshole. You can be called "unkind," "unyogic," or have your actions labelled "not spiritual" and still be a good human being that follows the guidelines of yoga and spirituality. When you have set clear, fair, and compassionate boundaries and the receiver has a negative reaction it's not your burden to bear.

Finally, if you find yourself accidentally being a spiritual asshole there's no need to impose more of the same comparison or judgement on yourself. Dwelling on the past will never change the present circumstances. Make amends to those you've hurt if you can, resolve to do better, and move forward with your best, radiant self.

The whole idea of the "spiritual asshole" highlights the importance of using the values of yoga and energetic work to uplift and inspire as this belief system was never meant to drag anyone down, only to enhance the lives of anyone open to receiving the teachings. Through these lessons we are reminded of our potential for good so that we make a positive impact and foster meaningful connections in our relationships.

7

CHAKRA ROAD MAP

Before the age of Google Maps, as a kid I was very proud to be the navigator on some of our family road trips. Glancing over road maps to see how everything was connected was special; it was like being able to see the future. You could look on the map, find turnoffs on your route and "poof" they appeared right in front of your eyes.

Chakras are like road maps for the soul. They tip you off with messages and warnings all the time. This is great if you understand how to decode the map, but what if it's completely foreign? By learning the signs and signals of your map, you'll never miss another turnoff again.

Understanding the role of energy in a yoga practice is the 1st step to your chakra road map. Working with our energetic field speaks to what energy can do for us—and what it cannot do. Becoming aware of our energetic presence is empowering. It's like being given a different lens to see the world in a whole new light. As we practice, feel, experience, and trust, we gain knowledge of how everything really "works" rather than what is seen on the surface. This opens us up to new possibilities.

Some days, it might feel like a burden but never forget that energy is always used for our greatest good—the universe will never bring you anything that you're not ready for. When energy is used responsibly, it is a gift. Seeking to understand that gift is necessary to unlock its potential. The following quote seems to sum it up perfectly.

> "Your anger? It's telling you where you feel powerless. Your anxiety? It's telling you that something in your life is off balance. Your fear? It's telling you what you care about. Your apathy? It's telling you where you're overextended and burnt out. Your feelings aren't random, they are messengers. And if you want to get anywhere, you need to be able to let them speak to you and tell you what you really need."
>
> - Breanna Wiest

This message speaks volumes about how to embrace the emotions that come up which are deemed as "negative." These signals are coming up for a reason! They are there to guide you towards the version of yourself you deserve to be. Pushing down or casting out these hints won't do you justice. Instead, ask "Why is this coming up in the first place?"

These emotions can get stored in specific places in the body. The energetic "hot spots" in eastern philosophy are known as the chakra system, meant to govern specific areas of the body. When energy gets stuck or stagnant, your energetic field will start ringing alarm bells. The messages coming up are sent straight to your intuition. If you don't listen, that's when the body gets louder to the point that you can't ignore it anymore—forming disease or dysfunction.

In a yoga practice, we can apply this lesson to how we deal with what comes up on the mat. When an emotional experience or memory floats into our consciousness, it likely resurfaced for a reason. Rather than disengaging through struggle and rejection, perhaps it is time to feel, breathe, then finally let it go—coming back into the present through body and breath.

When we cope with challenges in this way, it "lightens the load" energetically. Through this method we go from being a puppet with strings—completely powerless—to being able to see the strings and over time, cut the cords that bind us. Suddenly, those triggers that once caused so much turmoil might not have the same sting.

By this point, hopefully you are on board with how our energetic presence and receptivity impacts our life. The question on most lips is not the faith of what energy can do, it's "What can energy NOT do?" Answering this question involves acceptance of the fact that it is not a hard "yes" or a hard "no" in terms of the outcome of energetic work. Our faith and beliefs around energy affect efficacy. If the immediate reaction is "This is bullshit but I'll try it anyway," it will leave very little impression vs. "I am curious and open to what I will receive."

These two statements hold significantly different potential. The first statement would be like inviting someone over for tea but instead of welcoming them in with an open door, you make them go through a hardcore obstacle course before entering your house—they might not even make it to the first step, let alone make it into your home. Holding a polarized belief about energy—or being somewhere in between—will have a direct effect on what you receive. I have watched miracles and I have seen flops when it comes to energetic work.

We must take responsibility for our circumstances and mindset. The other factor is whether you are truly ready to "do the work." So, what is meant by "doing the work?" To better grasp this concept, let's take a closer look at how ideas or thought are manifested into reality.

Look at what's around you right now. Take note of what you're sitting on, what you're wearing, any devices, structures, or furniture. Every single thing that has been created was once thought. These were all the figment of someone's imagination being manifested before they were built into something tangible. How crazy is that?! Even if you are outside, laying on the grass, with nothing to see but trees, sky, birds, and animals in the forest—arguably, these were all born out of the ether at some point. Created by some divine "spark" of energy that formed the universe as we know it.

That spark is just as important as the willingness to build. This point can be illustrated further by using Tarot cards as an example. Reading tarot cards is a way of gaining clarity and insight into past, present, and future situations—acting as a mirror to the soul. In a reading, the Star is part of the major arcana to suggest major life shifts, typically representing the "spark" or the inspiration that makes miracles happen.

Although this card is very favourable, to see anything materialize from that spark requires something tangible to bring it into reality. Without something to "ground" that inspiration, it stays stuck in the ether, waiting to be manifested. This implies that action is required to make the magic happen. There have been so many ideas left in the ether, just waiting for their moment! How many times have you heard yourself or someone else say "I want to start a business," or "I'd love to travel," or "I'm going to finally do _____ which I've always wanted to do" but it never seems to happen?

The act of "doing the work" has many implications in our life and spiritual practice, but the essence of this concept lies in the willingness to take actionable steps forward. Like the old saying goes, "Rome wasn't built in a day" and neither were anyone's dreams.

So how is this idea of "doing the work" applied to our energetic receptivity? It is our willingness to look at our life with just as much attention and care as our yoga practice—recognizing that the two might not be so different after all. If these revelations come up on the mat, but they get ignored the minute they come up in "real life" situations, then is the work really being done? If healing is the request, it must be done holistically—our energetic practice on the mat is not meant to be a band-aid.

"Quick fixes" are like using duct tape for heavy machinery—sooner or later you'll have to deal with the consequences. True healing involves looking at all the factors—our life, relationships, emotions, blocks, and patterns that seem to keep coming up. Mending these facets of life will be the glue that holds everything together. Forming that "glue" may require additional support. Doing the work means more than just getting on the mat and being self-reflective, healing these other areas of life might mean getting help.

There's nothing wrong with seeing a doctor, osteopath, counsellor, physiotherapist, nutritionist, acupuncturist or whoever else you feel will support you in living your best life. Having these professionals as a support system is invaluable to your health and even spiritual growth! No one's path to healing is linear and not a single person's path is the same.

What might "work" for one person as a solution will not even make a dent in the problem for someone else. Balancing allopathic medicine with alternative approaches can prompt serious breakthroughs. With these decisions on treatment, each experience is unique. Although yoga can create space for miracles, there are more pieces to the puzzle.

We must take responsibility for the needs of the body, mind, and spirit which require a holistic approach—using eastern and western methodology. The two are meant to complement each other rather than antagonize. Dancing, nature, therapy, or even tea with a good friend can all be included in that prescription. It is up to each of us to discover what heals the body and ignites the soul.

On this path to discovery, soul seekers tend to have a deep desire to open every chakra. If you've been closed off for a long time, then hauling ass in the other direction seems like the right answer. The fact is that empathy, vulnerability, and energy all need a safe container that requires balance. Being too far on either end of the spectrum is a recipe for disaster.

This is the reason why, when sequencing, we wouldn't want to practice ALL heart openers or ALL twists for the entire practice. Not to mention the physical repercussions of only opening certain tissues and neglecting others. With most things in life, balance is key and the work we do on the mat is no exception.

The good news is that energy goes to where it needs to flow, meaning that if one area is meant to "open" a certain chakra, if that space is already open, it will seek to find balance instead. In addition, opening or balancing doesn't have to be related to physical sensation. Energy can also be supported through breath and intention. When we intentionally send energy, breath, affirmations, or visualisations into that "spot" we can break up whatever is blocking us from being balanced. Energy can move into a completely different chakra when the focus is shifted—applying the strength of intention in a whole new way.

Never underestimate the power of your intention. We are only energy. Energy cannot be destroyed, only shifted into a completely new form. We are the creators of our own masterpiece. It is us, in a relationship with the universe, co-creating the beauty that is our life.

With the recognition that we have power—yet ultimately no control—it's easy to see how the events that unfold are happening for our benefit rather than our damnation. If we can switch the conversation to "What can I learn from this experience?" We go from a state of powerlessness to seeing the puppet strings. The true chakra road map comes with time and practice so that we can see how this divine plan all comes together.

8

MULADHARA

THE ROOT OR 1ST CHAKRA

I grew up on Vancouver Island, part of coastal British Columbia in Canada. My parents reinforced the values that made this a heavenly place to explore for me and my sisters, raising us to respect and appreciate the world around us. I have many fond memories of playing in the forest, swimming in the ocean, hanging out on beaches, jumping into rivers and lakes on hot summer days, and shredding on a snowboard. Being connected to nature was a part of me that resonated deeply with my soul.

When I attended university in Vancouver, settling into an urban lifestyle was surprisingly easy. It was a city still relatively connected to the outdoors with mountains, oceans, and forests which was what probably made the transition feel seamless. In addition to plenty of greenspace, especially around the campus itself, the university had clubs dedicated to the activities I loved including yoga and snowboarding. For a city and an education, it was a perfect match.

I was studying Kinesiology so that I could apply for a competitive masters program. I remember studying morning to night in the hopes of better grades. I had the pre-requisites memorized, even the percentages I needed to get accepted. The stress ate away at me. When my final exams were finished, I would be violently ill for days. I neglected my personal care and basic needs to try to keep up. When I looked at the path I was going down, the question came up, "Is this what I really want?"

Getting into this masters program meant that I could do meaningful work and have a sustainable career path which seemed like the practical thing to do. I wondered if I had to keep torturing myself so that I could eventually be happy. Could I fulfill both needs without sacrificing myself in the process? When I reflected on what I really wanted, I couldn't stop thinking about everything I was passionate about. Life didn't feel complete without yoga, snowboarding, and being out in nature. No other circumstances made me happier.

It was around this time that I was introduced to a friend who lived in Whistler. My first visit there, I had the time of my life and thought, "one day, I'm going to live here!" I wasn't too sure how I was going to make this happen. I hadn't finished school yet, so the thought crossed my mind that maybe I'd find temporary work and do a season. I already felt like Whistler was home, I just needed to put roots down.

I began crashing on my friend's couch regularly which lead me to wonder, "where's all the yoga?" I was surprised there weren't a lot of options in town, especially in the village which is where most people gather for access to the shops, lifts, and events. At the time, I wasn't a yoga teacher but I'd been practicing for many years with the dream of one day doing a teacher training. I was a broke student who prioritized school above everything else with my time and finances. I also questioned whether I could be a decent yoga teacher, even with the training. You had to be "good" at yoga to teach and I didn't feel like I fit the mold. I didn't think I'd ever be good enough.

Back in the city, in addition to the classes I was attending with my school's yoga club, I'd been attending a few classes at a local studio. I noticed on their website that they were hoping to open other studios in neighboring communities. I talked to my boyfriend who had been considering putting his savings into a business. When I mentioned the need for a studio in Whistler, his response was very supportive. I went out on a limb, emailing the studio to see if Whistler was in the cards.

Fortunately, the woman who replied, Helene Whitfield, was very open to the idea. She was a wonderful mentor who taught me so much. I will always be grateful for her guidance, especially the day she casually mentioned, "We'll get you into the next yoga teacher training." I was stunned. Me? A yoga teacher? I couldn't even do a headstand, let alone a handstand. I wondered who would want to take classes from me—all my fears came to the surface. The same stories kept playing in my head that questioned whether I was "good enough" to do any of this. Become a yoga teacher and a studio owner? It seemed like such a far reach. Despite the negative thoughts that surfaced, I knew in my heart it was the right decision. I am so grateful for that initial nudge from her to take the journey that I'd secretly craved for nearly a decade.

When I moved up to Whistler, finished the training, and opened the studio, it was like everything began falling into place. I finally had a place where I felt like I belonged, for me this was "home." Soon after the studio opened, Helene and I ended our business relationship on good terms which meant I was given the chance to grow the studio independently. I made plenty of mistakes along the way in those initial years even before we separated—it was very tough—but I never regretted knowing the foundation that fed my spirit. When I look back on the signs that I tuned in to, I knew I was supported throughout the whole experience, even during the hard parts.

There are a few reasons why I mention this story in the context of the 1st chakra, Muladhara. This energetic space is the foundation for all other chakras—it governs our basic needs consistent with security, survival, instinct, and sense of belonging. When I was looking to "set my roots," I had a strong sense of who I was, and I knew "home" before I had even lived there. The qualities that enable you to know yourself on a deeper level are essential to create stability and balance energetically.

Without meeting our basic needs, we are unable to ascend spiritually since all focus needs to shift towards survival. Fulfilling the needs of Muladhara does not need to be glamorous—a roof over your head, a warm bed, feeling supported by your loved ones, and a consistent source of nourishing food will do the trick. It doesn't matter whether a person lives in a home with a dirt floor or a million dollar mansion, both individuals have the potential to construct a strong 1st chakra. Although there may be external circumstances influencing this energetic space, mindset plays a major role in its development. Feeling like there's never enough to go around will rob this energetic center of its power.

Hoarding and always focusing on "what's mine" and "How can I come out on top?" reeks of the fear that feeds the feelings of insufficiency. This mindset seeks to fill a non-existent void. When there's always a desire to purchase a bigger home, a nicer car, or the latest gadget, it's tied to a sense of scarcity that stems from the need for security. There's nothing wrong with wanting these things, given that it's not tied into a toxic mindset.

Often the urge to fill this sense of longing has a deeper meaning whether that's linked to pleasing others, attempting to cure emotional emptiness, or avoiding feelings of inadequacy. Far too many people use the accumulation of wealth to mask the pain they feel. Accumulating more "stuff" might bring about happiness temporarily but a return to "wholeness" will never happen without a serious mindset shift. Especially since the feeling of "lack" keeps attracting that same scarcity energetically, perpetuating a cycle that blocks abundance.

At one time, the mindset of "lack" ensured survival. The fear of not having shelter, food, or other basic needs to survive prompted our ancestors to create stability. In modern society, usually these basics are met, yet the fear of not having enough still feels like a threat. To get rid of this damaging belief once and for all, we must concentrate on what we already have—gratitude being the medicine that invites more blessings. The first step to getting out of this thought pattern is catching yourself in it. When I began recognizing my misguided beliefs, I started releasing myself from my fears. This can be around love, money, success, or anything else that you "think" is lacking.

Henry Ford once said, "Whether you think you can or you can't, you're right." As corny as it sounds, he is 100% right. The minute we tell ourselves "there's not enough money" or "I don't belong," the universe will send us signs and signals that will prove our bias. Luckily, when we look for opportunity, positivity, gifts, and abundance, we'll find those will show up too.

To make this magic happen, reframing incorrect thoughts is a great place to start. For example, regarding negative financial biases, an affirmation like "I am a money magnet," "money flows to me easily," or "there's always enough to go around" can create miracles, big and small. When I started to heal my thoughts about money, I would receive little surprises as confirmation—like finding $20 on the street here, or an unexpected work opportunity there. I realized I was the conductor when it came to creating the foundation to thrive. Now the skeptics out there may automatically jump to say, "Hey, finding $20 is not manifesting. It's just luck."

Before you completely write it off, consider this: if you open yourself up to the possibility—even for a second—that you could manifest these opportunities, perhaps you are allowing more awareness to come through so that these gifts appear in the right moment. For instance, if $20 was lying on the sidewalk while you are thinking intensely about your day, you might walk right past it, but if you are clear and filled with joy, then perhaps your openness makes you more observant so you spot that bill on the ground. Whether you are fully on board with this idea of manifesting or not, there are more possibilities that appear when we are open and present.

This idea of having openness and being present can play a powerful role in how life "plays out." When we tap into these qualities, it's easier to receive little signals that guide us back to our true selves, or the basis of our identity. In the story of how I ended up in Whistler, my choices were centered around identity. I knew instantly Whistler was "home" even when it was only my first visit. This deep and confident "knowing" is like the old saying that you can "feel it in your bones."

Being given an intense, unquestionable, unexplainable urge to follow through based on this "knowing" is a form of divine guidance—like a compass pointing us back on the right path. This skill blossoms from knowing who you are and what you stand for. Although an argument could be said that it is purely intuition—which does tie in since the 1st chakra is the foundation for intuition to be built upon—there is something deeper, more primal even.

When you understand and acknowledge your roots, you know where you come from and where you're going. With this stability, there's no confusion about the answers to life's big questions since deep down, this "knowing" has already given a clear message. The problem is, there are many circumstances in life that make us "forget" who we are. Negative experiences create imprints that block the ability to understand our true self. This often leads to a desire to "fill in the gaps." With the tangible, earthy quality of the 1st chakra, attempting to fill this void could look like excessive shopping habits, hoarding, or the acquisition of more and more "things." These "fillers" never create the foundation, only meaningful experiences related to identity can bridge that gap.

Identity is shaped by culture, personality, and upbringing. Family plays a big role in the development of identity, including systems of beliefs. For instance, negative biases may have been formed early on from witnessing family struggles around money, love, shelter, or other basic needs. These moments are a demonstration of how to function in the "real world" as adults.

Unfortunately, these aren't always healthy patterns to replicate. It's easy—and very Freudian—to blame our parents for everything wrong with us but it's more complicated than that. Parents are also the many things that are right with us! When I look back on my own childhood, there were times I learned bad habits that I've had to heal as an adult. However, there were also many moments when I was taught values—directly and indirectly—that brought me to where I am today thanks to my wonderful, loving, and supportive parents. If your parents ever made a mistake, they are only human! Just like you and me.

They did the best they could with what they had. Although that doesn't condone their actions, it can shed some light on the path to forgiveness so that you can move on. No matter what situations were present growing up, it is our job to take responsibility for our circumstances.

Marie Forleo affirms, "Despite what society, your family, or your mind have led you to believe, you are not broken. Nothing is intrinsically wrong with you." No matter what we've been fed, we have the power to make changes. It's never too late to uncover the parts of yourself that aren't "you"—or what no longer resonates with who you've become. Shedding those layers is a way of tapping into who you truly are.

So how do we create change when there's a feeling of being "stuck"? Mindset is a great start—what's the next step? Striding in the right direction means remembering the true self before all the other gunk got in the way. Healing for the 1st chakra means getting to know the self intimately. Meditation is known as the ultimate cure as being able to sit comfortably with yourself is extremely intimate. Without distractions it's just you—and occasionally the universe—communicating wholeheartedly. This can be scary!

If meditation is new to you, the idea of being left alone with your thoughts potentially running wild is terrifying. Mantras can be useful for leaning into stillness by creating a point of focus. The affirmation, which can be repeated as a mantra, for the 1st chakra is "I am." "I am" can be used to call in whatever you want to reaffirm in your life. Keep it away from labels like "I am a parent" or "I am my career" as these labels aren't inherently who you are on a deeper level. The roles we play aren't needed for this exercise, only the qualities we want to embody to step into our full potential. These are just a few examples of how "I am" statements can be used:

I am powerful

I am beautiful

I am abundant

I am bliss

I am strong

I am calm

I am stable

The potential is endless for "I am" statements. Once, a student asked me "But what if you don't believe what you're telling yourself?" In some way, if there's an "I am" statement that's popping into your head, your soul must believe it on some level. Even if it's the tiniest belief imaginable. With repetition, that new set of beliefs becomes your reality. We reinforce whatever thoughts we repeat the most. With repetition, the neural networks of the brain are strengthened and constructed—what scientists refer to as "neuroplasticity."

That is how we can be hardwired for beliefs through our brain and nervous system. When we default to positive, reaffirming thoughts, we destroy the pathways that drag our spirit down—they grow weak and eventually fade. Suddenly, these "I am" statements ground you in your true nature and what you're capable of. Even when it seems like a stretch, trust yourself. You know your roots, you know who you are when you clear out the bullshit. Don't let doubt come in and take that away from you. Let those "I am" statements flow organically and watch the magic happen. One unexpected side effect of this exercise is the realization that you already embody all of the qualities you seek—sometimes we just need to re-confirm that they are present.

Lastly, not everyone will appreciate your transformation when you commit to making changes that affect your identity. Some prefer that you play small or hold onto those patterns that have held you back. Plus, those around you are used to the "old you"—where friends or family are concerned, there might be a bit of an adjustment period. Suddenly, the old triggers become less of a switch or old relationships need to be renegotiated. Resist the temptation to fall back into old patterns. The minute we commit to doing something different, there might be little spiritual "tests."

For example, when I made the decision to quit drinking, I'd have friends of family who would say "just one drink?" Or "how about just this one time?" Rather than get upset or question myself, the clear answer was "no" or "no thanks." Eventually, those questions stop. Never be scared to reveal the true "you" in these situations. Those who love and care for you will still be there and those who don't appreciate your authenticity will fall by the wayside.

Clearly seeing our origins helps us commit to our inner "knowing"—giving us the keys to see the true self. If we know where we've come from, then we also know what direction to take. We don't have to have a "pretty" upbringing by any means to promote deep and stable roots. By devoting yourself to a healthy mindset, clearing out the clutter that isn't you, and taking responsibility for the circumstances, you have will effectively built a strong foundation to grow from which is what the 1st chakra is all about.

POSTURES THAT CAN HELP SUPPORT MULADHARA

These are a few postures that support (but are not limited to) the 1st chakra:

- Meditation
- Savasana
- Supported Child's Pose
- Legs up the wall
- Supported Forward Fold

9

SVADHISTHANA
THE SACRAL OR 2ND CHAKRA

Taking the leap into entrepreneurship as a yoga studio owner was one of the toughest yet most rewarding decisions I've ever made. The question of whether it would end up "working out" merged with strong hopes and dreams, gave rise to a complicated rollercoaster of emotions. I accredited my sanity to the deep connection I had to my intuition and spirit through yoga and mindfulness, especially on the tough days.

Despite the waves of emotion and fear I experienced through the process, I knew deep in my heart that this act of service in my community would become wildly successful—I had the sense that this studio and its teachers would touch the lives of many people for years to come. This was part of the driving force that kept me grounded during the challenges faced over the first few years after the studio opened.

When it comes to emotional upheaval—and emotions or feelings in general—there is a strong connection to the 2nd chakra, Svadhisthana, located at the pelvis. With the physical manifestation of emotional well-being it's important to revisit the role of the nervous system, an integral element of restorative yoga, and how it reacts under stress.

From an evolutionary perspective, the fight-or-flight response becomes active during stressful situations thereby preparing someone to fight off an attacker or flee from the situation, both actions fueled by the instinct for self-preservation and survival.

For many people this is "turned on" in moments that are not related to life-or-death matters, and stays in full force for an inappropriate amount of time, even after the initial threat has subsided. This has a negative consequence on health and well-being. This preparation to fight or flee has a direct effect on musculoskeletal function considering which muscles are used to execute these actions. The muscles that perform hip flexion and extension can be negatively impacted by the fight-or-flight response along with muscles of the leg.

This is one of the reasons tension can occur around the pelvis, particularly for the psoas, gluteal muscles, and muscles that perform synergist actions during running. This area is also particularly challenging for active people, including runners or bikers, as it's often an area that gets overused. This makes focusing on the muscles around the pelvis more important than ever for those who experience stress or high levels of activity on a regular basis.

In the face of the stress I experienced with opening the studio, I also felt a great deal of joy. This was an opportunity to live my "dharma"—commonly referred to as my calling—through serving others by providing a sacred space. Before we opened our doors, I fondly remember a friend mentioning in anticipation, "wow, it's almost like you're having a baby!" Creating this community was like a birth—the birth of a new chapter that brought a whole new set of experiences, responsibilities, and fulfillment. Although the second chakra has a clear relationship with literal birth since the pelvis is home to our reproductive organs, it also shares a strong link with creativity—the ability to give life to new ideas.

For me, the yoga studio began as a dream which was then manifested into reality. Each of us has the potential to birth the life we truly want through the choices we make. We have the power to take that dream job, travel the world, stay in a relationship, leave a relationship, or make the changes necessary to thrive. The lower chakras tend to be associated with our sense of stability, they are the basis for who we are and how we see ourselves—therefore it can be challenging to overcome fears associated with the 2nd chakra. Recognizing our own power to produce change isn't always easy, especially if it's a pattern that we've been comfortable in for a while.

I had been vegetarian for about 15 years and throughout that journey I had considered transitioning to being vegan. I already felt that my diet was challenging at times so I was hesitant to make what felt like a major shift. I figured doing "something" as a vegetarian was better than nothing at all. I stayed complacent even though I didn't fully feel that my values were being honoured through my actions.

One year during the late winter I contracted a nasty bout of bronchitis. With sleepless nights due to breathing difficulties I was so desperate to get better that I was willing to try anything to support my healing. I began to research what caused bronchitis—I knew getting to the root of the issue could kick-start my recovery. Inflammation seemed to be one of the biggest triggers.

During this healing process that lasted many months and involved continuous self-reflection, I took a long, hard look at my diet. I considered what could contribute to inflammation or ameliorate it. As a vegetarian I always loved milk, cheese, and yogurt. These foods were often linked with inflammation, prompting me to give them up since I was eager to try anything to improve my situation. I always thought letting go of these foods would be the hardest part yet it was surprisingly easy.

I had built up excuses in my head for so long that it prevented me from the possibilities that were easily within my reach. Rather than this being a lesson about the value of being vegan, I consider it a lesson in connecting to your truth and overcoming stagnant patterns. The 2nd chakra loves and embraces change with its fluid-like nature.

Openness to transformation in many different forms—perspective shifts, aging, lifestyle changes, or major life shifts—will allow for buoyancy in this chakra that loves going with the flow. This ability to "go with the flow" and experience the emotions of life without attachment suddenly becomes natural and effortless. One of my experiences that helped me recognize an ability to "go with the flow" happened at an unexpected time.

My husband Kevin and I were visiting one of our favourite breakfast spots. When we walked back to our car, I noticed that one of our back passenger windows had been smashed. When I pointed it out, he saw that some of our belongings had been stolen. Silence accompanied the initial shock, then a long sigh. We began figuring out the steps that were necessary in this situation. Both of us remained calm and collected as we created a plan of action. After the ordeal was over Kevin mentioned, "I'm really impressed with how we handled that. I don't think we could've done that 10 years ago."

Kevin was right, we had stayed cool as a cucumber throughout the whole situation despite it being disappointing, time consuming, and an unexpected expense. Strong emotions never took hold long enough to distract us from the task that would support us in moving forward. In this difficult scenario there was a moment of surrender with an acknowledgement that this was part of some divine flow. Perhaps this inconvenience had a lesson to teach us.

One of the most surprising facets of this interaction was the reaction I had towards the perpetrator who was never found. Rather than anger or hate, my initial reaction was one of compassion. I wondered, "What could drive someone to do this?"

I was curious as to what kind of life this person led and how desperate they must be to commit this crime. I imagined someone who had had a rough childhood leading them down a path towards crime, drugs, and delinquency. Although this image may not be an accurate representation of reality, it gave me a sense of understanding about why someone might make these choices.

Although compassion is often associated with the heart chakra, it shares an important role to svadhistana. Our ability to connect on an emotional level to other beings that share this planet will greatly influence the health of the 2nd chakra. This deep sense of compassion, understanding, and awareness is a key part of the healing process on an energetic level. To experience any form of self-actualization, nurturing our sense of compassion is essential towards other people and ourselves.

The relationship we create with the person staring back at us in the mirror is the most important connection we will ever have. It will influence how we see the world and our connections to everyone in it. Personal relationships play a major role in the flow of the 2nd chakra. Due to its relevance regarding sex organs and birth, its value to intimate relationships cannot be understated—particularly romantic partners but also friendships and even acquaintances.

When reflecting on your network involving the people closest to you, observe the relationship you have with yourself first. By actively practicing acts of love and kindness towards yourself, this energy will be reflected through your personal relationships. What I've noticed in my own life and practice is that the superficial relationships I held onto in my earlier life have fallen to the wayside.

Now, I have an abundance of caring, loving connections who appreciate and uplift me. Having a positive inner circle does not mean that you will never have disagreements with your loved ones, but you share common ground and hold a deep respect for one another. This is the same respect that you have for yourself that you in turn send out into the world with your presence.

Having this awareness of the relationship with ourselves is a significant advantage in a restorative practice. The deep sense of compassion and understanding fostered through this relationship directly translates to the practice, ultimately transforming the way we treat ourselves when it comes to being truly comfortable. Having this principle as a priority will enhance any restorative practice on a physical and energetic level.

Sensation, feelings, and particularly pleasure are closely linked to the 2nd chakra. Those with a creative outlet, specifically anyone keen to bring their ideas to life, are more likely to experience harmony in this energetic space. It really is no surprise that artists and musicians usually have a very strong link with Svadhisthana to release their creative, sexual, and emotional energy. To foster growth in the 2nd chakra is to release untapped creative potential, pleasure, and joy. Sensation and the ability to feel deeply is at the heart of these experiences, making it a hot topic when it comes to restorative yoga.

Allowing discomfort to persist in order to preserve someone else's comfort is a cultural norm, especially when that person is in a place of authority. In yoga, it becomes easy to question the innate intelligence of the body when a yoga teacher offers a suggestion that creates pain or discomfort. Many students are concerned that practicing a different shape or questioning their teacher will come off as disrespectful or arrogant. Shifting this paradigm is necessary for a healthy student-teacher relationship. I'd like to think that teaching is a conversation—it does not work when it is one sided—as a teacher, we can only understand sensations through the body we've been given. The conversation begins when the student shares their truth through their expression of the practice.

Since we can't begin to comprehend what it's like to live in someone else's body, yoga teachers or health professionals can assist, but ultimately, each person knows their own body the best.

With the intention of restorative yoga, it is our duty to honour our body's signals—taking action in these circumstances starts with recognizing what's problematic. In restorative yoga, this is what blocks you from bliss. When your mind focuses more on the sensation—whether it's stretching, pain, sharpness, dullness, tingling or otherwise—then it takes you out of that moment of bliss. Empowerment is the ability to choose absolute freedom through comfort. This means that you may have to use more props than the person next to you or practice a different pose altogether.

Choosing to care less about what other people think is liberating. When we tune into the sensations of our body, it separates us from the distractions that aren't allowing us to hold space for ourselves, which include internalized patterns of judgement or shame. Experiencing pleasure and bliss means having the confidence and bravery to take the variations, props, and suggestions that work with the sensations that arise.

While writing this book I considered how I was showing up in my own life with bravery and confidence. Although these are values I vehemently stand with, one story kept rearing its ugly head that I resisted telling—an experience I've barely shared with anyone. Like a physical wound that requires healing, the road to recovery often demands revisiting the pain.

This emotional vulnerability supports the essence of the 2nd chakra. When we feel ready to break down the walls that have been built up, it creates space for healing—sharing and connecting authentically is part of that process. It is my hope that in communicating this story, it builds an authentic connection with those who have also been impacted by similar circumstances in regards to sexual trauma.

During college in early spring I was invited out to a club with some friends. I had arranged to meet them downtown in a specific location so I could leave my phone at home. When I arrived at the venue I had very little money as a broke student, and I was also tipsy from drinking at home so I wouldn't have to buy anything from the bar. I searched tirelessly for my friends, eventually hopping from bar to bar downtown hoping to find them out somewhere else. At one of the clubs I bumped into someone I knew, a guy I'd gone on a date or two with, who I'd met at my part-time job. We danced, flirted, and he introduced me to his friends—at this point I'd given up on trying to find mine.

When I was ready to head out he offered to walk with me. It was an extremely cold night with snow still on the ground, and with less than $10 in my pocket I figured it was my best option. On the hour-long walk I remember him making sexual jokes and innuendo towards me. My response was to make it clear that I was not having sex with him. At 18 years old I'd had a few boyfriends previously but I'd never gone "all the way" with anyone. Instead, I had consciously chosen to wait for the right person.

When I arrived home he came downstairs to my suite, I let him into my bed. I liked him, I wanted to make out but I told him multiple times I didn't want to have sex. He began taking off my clothes. I was drunk. There were certain acts I felt comfortable to do but he relentlessly pushed my boundaries. Finally, in a moment of complete clarity like I had been "snapped" sober, I put my hand over my vagina to say, "I am not having sex with you."

I cannot even remember if he replied but I do remember my shame and disgust when he entered me. I lay there, not knowing what to do. I felt completely powerless, I even wondered if I should just lay there and enjoy it. The following morning, I drove him home then texted him later that day, thinking maybe if we tried dating it would make everything feel ok. I never spoke to him again.

After that I cried every day for weeks, I felt like a piece of garbage. The power of choice had been ripped away, filling me with rage and sadness. During our darkest times, the universe tends to listen more closely, sending us angels that show up at exactly the right time. The universe must have heard my prayers. For me, my angel arrived about a month later in the form of the man who would become my husband. Although this divine timing would not heal this deep wound, his love and support showed me that I could trust again.

Sexual abuse can greatly disturb the power and potency of the 2nd chakra, in my experience it left only darkness and despair. I yearned to "numb" out the feelings associated with the trauma; my vice was usually alcohol or anything else distracting me from the pain. Louise

Hay adds that those who experience this form of trauma tend to want to protect themselves. One of the coping mechanisms she refers to is weight gain, an unconscious pattern of choices that are meant to defend against current or future abusers.

These strategies to cope are distractions from the potential to heal. Instead of using substances, food, or any other distraction, it is our calling to come back to who we truly are. Each path to healing is unique yet we must never lose sight that it begins with self-love and acceptance. With yoga—in combination with therapy, energy work, alternative health methods, support from those you trust, and other healthy patterns—we can be reminded of these fundamental ideals, lifting us up even when we feel forced down. Yoga and energy work taps into the true potential of the 2nd chakra to combat numbness, and act as a reminder of the beauty to discover through feeling and experiencing.

Anger, sadness, or intensity are bound to come up through this transition. These emotions are all perfectly healthy to flow through given that we are also willing to let them go.

Learning to let go might be one of the most difficult spiritual lessons, especially with pain and trauma. Letting go requires a great deal of patience with a willingness to revisit the issue until it doesn't hold the same heavy emotional weight. This can take years, even decades to fully process. Emotional trauma bears similarities with the healing process of a deep physical wound.

Although a gash will heal over eventually, there will always be a scar. That scar might feel uncomfortable when you run your finger over it, but it lacks the agony it once caused. Certain massage techniques or acupuncture may give it relief—just like how emotional wounds heal when we work on ourselves—but it will never fully disappear. Luckily, one of the gifts of the 2nd chakra is patience. When we pair that with radical acceptance, we can allow ourselves to approve of the broken, beautiful soul we were always meant to be.

POSTURES THAT CAN HELP SUPPORT SVADHISTHANA

These are a few postures that support (but are not limited to) the 2nd chakra:

- Reclined supported butterfly
- Supported seated angle pose
- Supported Child's Pose
- Reverse corpse pose - advasana

10

MANIPURA

THE SOLAR PLEXUS OR 3RD CHAKRA

At 12 years old I bought my first bikini, a rite of passage that felt exciting. I was proud to purchase the blue number on my own as a celebration of the woman I was becoming. Summer brought me so much joy—I was always obsessed with being in the water and hanging out in the sunshine, so naturally I couldn't wait to show off my new look.

At a local swimming spot, I was walking past a group of older boys on my way to the water. Out of the corner of my eye I saw one point at me to say, "there's the girl that's going to gain 20 lbs when she goes to college."

I could hear the other boys chuckling away. Thoughts of fear, disappointment, and humiliation ran through my mind. "What about my body would make them say that?" I wondered. "Was I already too fat for this bikini?"

My thoughts churned and I finally arrived at the conclusion that my body wasn't good enough for public consumption. I spent years trying to meet an unrealistic standard of beauty. Shortly after that incident, I remember trying to get through the day by eating only one apple or skipping dinners to go out with friends. This made me feel powerful and in control of my body which dulled out the negative commentary that infested my mind and drove me to feel shame.

I spent many years struggling with this mindset that was only reinforced by popular culture—from television to magazines—and the expectations of society weighing heavily. It did not help that there were other traumatic moments that reinforced the fears I felt, directly related to my body image. Comments made by strangers, relatives, and friends may seem harmless now but were detrimental growing up. This type of feedback regarding personal image directly influences the development of the 3rd chakra.

The energetic space located around the navel known as the 3rd chakra or Manipura typically develops during adolescence into early adulthood. For me, this upsetting moment in time represented the ushering in of my teenage years and the lens that I used to view myself. This experience was two-fold which very accurately depicts the positive and negative qualities associated with Manipura. I felt shame and disgust towards my body but when I performed actions to alleviate those feelings I would experience a sense of power and control as a result.

This personal power was through the approval that I sought from other people which left me feeling dissatisfied. I could never experience fulfillment since the true power of Manipura lies in the appreciation for yourself, not in the approval of others. This foundation linked to self-esteem is built for most people in adolescence. This makes it difficult to integrate due to the impact of bullying that happens all too often during grade school. I was all too familiar with this form of harassment.

One morning on the bus in high school, I overheard two people I barely knew sitting behind me, cracking jokes. I can't even remember what they said about me, I did my best to tune them out, but I remember the state of fear that settled in. At the age of sixteen I was no stranger to being bullied, it's something I had dealt with for most of my life by this point.

There was just something about this encounter that I sensed was different even as I tried to ignore it. I heard someone playing with a lighter, the flicking sound it made before it was lit. Then suddenly a "woosh" noise erupted and I felt heat behind my head. I heard the snickering from behind me but I didn't dare turn around.

When I arrived at school, I immediately rushed into the washroom and felt the back of my head. My hair had been set on fire. Running fingers over the stringy, singed hair made me feel hopeless and embarrassed. Something that I thought I had power and control over had been stripped away from me. I wondered what I had done to deserve this.

A study from Salmon & James wrote that 10% of secondary school-aged children reported being bullied "sometimes or more often" during their term while 4% were being victimized on a weekly basis. Victimisation at school may result in long-term social, emotional and psychological effects. It is no surprise that many children and teenagers carry these heavy burdens into adulthood.

Digestive problems, gut health, anxiety, self-esteem, and depression can originate in the 3rd chakra. This energetic space is fueled by inner strength, determination, and self-worth. Yoga—particularly styles that encourage body positivity—along with meditation, mindfulness, and affirmations can be a beautiful way of allowing this energetic powerhouse to flourish.

For me, this was a long journey. Looking back now, it almost feels like the thoughts and emotions of a completely different person. On the rare occasion, I still have "bad" days but my inner critic lacks the sting it once had—I can even laugh at in my mind by saying "that's a ridiculous thought" and carry on with my day. With new insight, I recognize that this inaccurate commentary holds no power.

With Manipura's connection to self-esteem, it should come as no surprise that personal power is a key ingredient to the health of this chakra. When my hair was set on fire, I instantly lost my sense of power. I also blamed myself, questioning what I could've done to stop it. At the time, I couldn't observe the obvious relationship to power the bullies were seeking. It was clear they were lacking power in their own life, perhaps at home or through their performance in school.

By attacking me, they could assert their dominance and feel as though they were taking back their power. Although this does not make up for what they did, I can look back on this incident and understand what may have motivated them to perform such a heinous act. It is through this understanding that I can also foster forgiveness and release my anger—an act of empowerment that will ultimately strengthen Manipura.

Concerns related to power can also be heavily involved with relationships to money. Greed, materialism, egotistical behavior, and narcissism all fall within 3rd chakra territory. In terms of money, those who experience imbalance will feel as though they never have enough, regardless of whether this is accurate.

Most people do indeed have everything they need provided to them—a roof over their head, access to food, water, healthcare, and more. However, there is an illusion that we must always be striving. A bigger house, a better car, nicer furniture, bigger and more expensive vacations. Longing for material wealth has negative consequences to emotional and spiritual well-being.

From early childhood I have a strong memory of walking past a cinnamon bun store in the mall. The smell of the freshly baked cinnamon buns with their creamy icing made me imagine how soft and delicious they must have been! I must have asked my mom a million times to stop for a cinnamon bun but we always rushed past. This gave me the impression that we could not afford to buy cinnamon buns despite that we always had our needs met—the price of cinnamon buns definitely was not a financial problem. Looking back on these circumstances, it's easy to understand there could've been a whole list of reasons why we never stopped for cinnamon buns —the amount of sugar they had or perhaps we were always running late—but my brain jumped to what seemed like the most logical conclusion: money, or lack of it.

To a child, this seemed like the piece that fit the puzzle even though it was far from the truth. My young mind picked up on other cues like receiving hand-me-down clothing or shopping at goodwill. I remember taking notice of some families going on vacations to exotic destinations in the summer when we would go camping. I grew up with the false belief that I had less than other people. This made me think I had to work extremely hard to feel fulfilled. On top of that, I had the need to hoard money, thinking it would ensure my success—I interpreted this as a path to avoid hardship.

This mentality towards wealth, funnily enough, did the opposite. I always felt like my finances could never catch up, as if there was never enough to go around. This feeling of "lack" blocked my ability to create financial freedom. It wasn't until my early twenties that I began to realize how destructive this thought pattern had been. This path to abundance has changed my relationship with money, wealth, and how I see life in general.

Contrary to popular belief, mostly created through media and cultural manipulation, abundance is not so far out of reach. In fact, many of us experience abundance very regularly! Gratitude is the medicine when feelings of "lack" are present. Pointing these moments of gratitude out in your mind can be very useful when cultivating an abundance mindset. This exercise is very powerful while in the moment—sipping tea, admiring a forest, watching snow fall, or the feeling of sand underneath your feet can all be done from a place of gratitude. True wealth is for those who can appreciate it and although some material goods are necessary to fulfil basic human needs, most desires go far beyond what's required for comfort and survival. Materialism gives a false sense of relief for those seeking abundance in the wrong places.

The illusion that with more belongings or by acquiring luxurious, expensive items, this will fill the void they experience. Over my lifetime, the deepest lessons in gratitude I've experienced involve concerns regarding my health and losing the people I care about. Health is needed to experience life fully—having an injury or health crisis may be a blessing in disguise. My injuries and health concerns have taught me compassion and provided me with clarity on gratitude. Suddenly, small acts like the ability to climb stairs become a blessing! Loss of a loved one on the other hand acts as an important reminder to have overwhelming gratitude for the people you love, who continue to show up in your life. At the end of the day, with mildly good health and loved ones present in some form—near or far—there is plenty to be grateful for.

One of the gifts I've always been grateful for is the ability to trust my gut, a vital characteristic of Manipura. This energetic space is responsible for processing in the literal sense, in terms of digestion, but it is also linked with how we assimilate emotionally and spiritually. Naturally, we will have signals through that experience of processing which offers insight into everything, from simple questions like "what should I be eating today to nourish myself?" to more complex concerns related to major life decisions. Leaning into those signals that connect us closer to true self will only bolster positive qualities of the 3rd chakra including confidence, inner strength, self-worth, and abundance.

Fear is an interesting signal to note in the gut. Have you ever had a fear that made you sick to your stomach? A lot of fears make the gut feel like it's tied up in knots. Fear is a survival tactic that likes to hang out in the lower chakras. Each chakra, 1 through 3, has a slightly different relationship to fear. The first chakra leans into the fears around survival and basic needs, the 2nd is related to relationships and the fluidity of life, while the 3rd speaks to fears around self-image and power. From the beginning of life to the end, we all experience fear—there's really no way around it. This is hardwired into our brain as part of our instinct. Rather than focusing on the impossible feat of destroying it, aim to move through it. Look that big scary "thing" in the face and do the thing—or don't do the thing and move on.

If you choose to "do the thing", the sense of relief afterwards—whether you soar or flop—is worth it. If you know it's not the right move, then make a solid decision and move on. This might leave you thinking, "but Emily, what if it's a BIG flop that I can't risk doing?" There's a road map for that. I've had people ask me before how I am so fearless in doing big things. The fact is, yes, I have fear but I don't let it stand in my way. My first reaction to fear is always "what's the worst that can happen?"

In 2008 I was accepted into a Bachelors program at a university that was tough to get into. I was so excited that I had "made the cut" and started planning my move to the city. By this point, I had already picked up and moved a few times—even sleeping out of my car on occasion—so I thought I could just find a place to live and everything would work out. Even with my best efforts, I ended up homeless for the first month of university. Now, "homeless" is a bit of a stretch, even though I didn't have a home, I was lucky enough to have friends in the city who would let me crash on their couch for a couple of days at a time.

Despite being broke, there were some cheap hostels to stay in when no one could host me. I no longer owned a car so there was zero "backup plan" but somehow, I made it work. This experience was my worst fear come to fruition. The idea of not having a home was terrifying! Yet I was so hell-bent on getting my education, I was even willing to sleep on a park bench if I had to. After this experience, I knew that I could handle anything. If living out of a small suitcase, discovering new transit routes every day, and scrambling to figure out my next place to sleep taught me anything, it's this: the strength of the human spirit. Through pure determination and will, I figured out how to move through my fear.

When fear was brought up again in 2012 while opening the studio, I just came back to the question "what's the worst that could happen?"

Well, both of us—me and my now husband—could end up homeless, but I knew that we would get through it. Of course, there's a spectrum of "worst case scenarios" and you might not always end up winning—but would you rather sit on the sidelines or actively participate in the magic unfolding in your life? It's better to lose and fail a hundred times than to not play at all—sometimes you need that many losses to get a big win. Fear is not something to be feared, rather it tells you what you are passionate about!

Questioning yourself with "what's the worst that could happen" could be your ticket to moving through that fear to get on the road to success—even if you fall off that road along the way. Stumbling is just one step on that journey. Perhaps those steps also include exciting "wins" leading us to consider the flip side of this question: "what's the best thing that could happen?!" Don't sell yourself short. We all deserve to make our dreams happen, one step at a time.

Although this story from university could arguably be a 1st chakra-related event, riding the wave of "not knowing" was an emotional experience that was processed through my gut. As home of the digestive system, the area of the 3rd chakra physically digests food but it also takes care of spiritual digestion. We process thoughts and emotions through this space energetically.

If you feel energetic constipation, the gut is where that flow gets stuck. So, what's going to get things moving again? From a yogic lens, we could use twists in a sequence and breathing that emphasizes the belly to release patterns of shame and guilt associated with the negative aspects of Manipura. Away from the mat, we could look at healthy ways of processing these emotions—resolving bottled up feelings can be done through tough conversations with whoever sparked the intensity, journaling about the experience, and using therapy to talk things through can all be effective methods of processing. These are just a few approaches to draw inspiration from. They are also examples of regaining personal power—a rewarding virtue of the 3rd chakra.

Rising into our personal power is an absolute gift. It helps us realize what we're truly capable of when we tear down the walls that have been built up by doubt, despair, and self-depreciation. As a teacher, there are many ways to empower students through their yoga practice.

Those who may not have power in their homes, at work, or with the people they encounter are suddenly gifted with the chance for complete autonomy. Don't want to practice this pose? *Then don't.* Want to use more props than everyone else? *Go for it.* This level of freedom, especially when it comes to encouraging comfort, is a foreign concept to most people. In a culture that is obsessed with making us uncomfortable, overworked, and overstimulated, relaxation is a form of rebellion. By exercising our right to choose, we step into our power, a strength that is accessed by nurturing Manipura.

POSTURES THAT CAN HELP SUPPORT MANIPURA

These are a few postures that support (but are not limited to) the 3rd chakra:

- Restorative twist over a bolster
- Reclined two knee twist
- Reclined one knee twist (with bolster or block support)
- 3 part breathing or deep belly breathing

11

ANAHATA

THE HEART OR 4TH CHAKRA

The day I lost my dad, I knew life would never be the same. Looking back on it now as an adult, it feels like a fucked-up dream. The process of losing him was greater than any pain I'd ever experienced, still to this day. It felt as though something within myself died but rather than burying this "thing," it stayed inside to rot. This dark, black sludge steeped inside me—a manifestation of emotional turmoil that literally made me feel sick.

I felt as though a limb had been hacked off and I was walking around, bleeding out, but no one on the outside noticed. At the time, I couldn't even imagine what functioning "normally" again would look like. Losing him as a teenager I had no idea how I'd get through the rest of life's big milestones but I knew somehow, I'd have to figure it out.

On this journey through the grieving process, I discovered a new "normal" so that every day would be a step forward. This slow and steady transition meant there was a transformation into something new. In an age where "being your best-self" is an esteemed goal, it may be risky to admit that creating a new-self may not be a shining, bright star. Instead, stands a humbled, beautiful mess.

"Joy and sorrow are inseparable… together they come and one sits alone with you… remember that the other is asleep upon your bed."

- Kahil Gibran

Loss is a great teacher. Eventually, we will lose everything: belongings, friends, family, and even our own body. This concept isn't meant to be terrifying, it's destined to liberate—if we realize our time is limited, then loving deeply is an obvious choice. To live by this principle is to enjoy freedom and clarity since living joyfully is our birthright.

Even with the pain and suffering that comes with human existence at our core, we are meant to experience joy and love fearlessly. These are the characteristics that define the heart chakra, Anahata. To fully embrace these qualities of love and joy, continually asking ones' self to stay "open" is essential.

When events happen that cause great loss, heartbreak, and despair, it may seem easier to close off from the world. This task of staying open isn't for the faint of heart. It requires deep trust and vulnerability. Trust that we're supported through the process of healing by a higher power and the vulnerability to recognize our own fragile human nature—more specifically, the tendency to avoid pain. This mechanism of pain avoidance is meant to protect us. However, emotional guarding can block the energetic space of the heart.

This prevents opportunities for love and joy to flourish. Recognizing when pain is blocking this chakra is the key to remaining open. There are some situations when guarding emotionally is a healthy and necessary action. Those who have overcome trauma in relationships would need to hold those walls high in certain situations. For example, when coming face-to-face with someone who is emotionally abusive, the act of setting firm boundaries cannot be understated. Using keen discernment is required when considering whether emotional guarding is helping or harming. In most cases, when shielding is the "default," it blocks our ability to live a joyous life filled with love and positive experiences.

When it comes to living joyously, many confuse this with the notion of "happiness." Both are wonderful emotions and yet the two are quite different. Usually, something external triggers happiness whereas joy is a state of being created internally. Happiness fluctuates with circumstances outside of our control while joy has a consistency since it is a conscious choice.

Although one might argue that you can choose to be happy, what I would suggest is that you are choosing joy instead. Happiness is a reaction whereas joy is a continuous state. Both are experiences that bring value into everyday life. Rather than demonize being happy, I am suggesting that when happiness diminishes, not to let it rob you of your joy. Joy is a soulful gift of the heart, one that should be used openly and often.

To live joyously means to free ourselves from the weights that drag us down. When we hold onto resentment, anger, and tension, this prevents us from tapping into joy. This is what makes forgiveness such an important piece of the puzzle when it comes to the matters of the heart. One aspect of forgiveness that confuses even the most prudent practitioners is the thought that forgiving someone condones their actions. Forgiving does not forgive the action itself, rather it sets you free from the poison of anger, hatred, and rage that you may feel towards the person who committed the act.

One proverb hits the nail right on the head, "holding onto anger is like drinking poison and expecting someone else to die." When we forgive and let go of the intensity, we feel that the person involved no longer holds any power over us. By releasing these emotions, we are cutting the ties that keep us connected to them. Each of us owes it to ourselves to have the freedom we deserve and forgiveness is the final step that makes this liberation possible. This might have you saying "but how do I do that?" Especially in situations that cut deeply.

Gabrielle Bernstein has some wise words on this topic. She suggests we do not even have to know "how" to forgive; we should instead focus on opening ourselves to recognize that we are ready for it. The idea is that when the door is open, the universe will help you step through it. Time and time again, miracles are made possible when we trust and surrender.

To have faith and surrender can seem impossible when significant loss is involved. Small tests of trust are a breeze compared to losing a career, a relationship, financial stability, or a loved one. It is no surprise that loss and forgiveness naturally weave together. When I experienced the loss of my dad, the grieving process showed me that even with all the love I felt, there was also intense anger. The anger I felt stemmed from the life choices he made that led him to get sick along with the sense of abandonment I felt towards his death.

Ultimately, I had to forgive him for being a human being with all of his flaws. I cannot expect perfection from him, or anyone, including myself. This understanding leads to another beautiful quality of the heart chakra: compassion.

When my dad passed away, I was already going through enough emotional turmoil as a teenager. Grief added a whole new layer to who I was becoming. During this period, there were times that I tried to hide the dark, gritty parts of myself. What I didn't realize was the need for expression of this darker side in healthy ways—I ignored that aspect of my existence which desperately needed to be embraced, loved, and sent compassion. Modern yoga can also be very good at disregarding the nefarious side of our nature as human beings.

The current philosophy tends to glorify the positive, bubbly facets of the yoga practice but completely rejects the notion that spirituality and anything in the universe seeks balance. It is imperative that every yoga practitioner sees beauty, brightness, and light but they should also gain a firm understanding of their dark side. In fact, making "friends" with this dark side can assist in spiritual awakening. Rather than indulging in the wills of this darker version of yourself, become fully prepared to call it out on its shit—just like you would a good friend. This creates a brighter path to truly see who you are and the direction you're heading.

At the time, rather than send love and compassion to this darker version of myself, I chose to cope in other ways. Some were healthy—yoga and sports for example—while others were downright destructive: binge drinking, partying, and anything that could numb out the heartbreak I felt. None of these things are inherently damaging if done responsibly, but I sought to be reckless to fill the hole in my heart. Unfortunately, none of these things could fill this void. In fact, nothing can. Under these circumstances, it only offered me the chance to grow, become stronger, and to learn to appreciate the love still present in my life.

Energetically, the heart craves to live openly. We all have the innate need to love and be loved. However, there are many circumstances in life that cause this energetic space to close off. This event could involve heartbreak, trauma, loss, or pain. For instance, those who have overcome significant loss or trauma can feel overwhelmed by even the smallest backbend. The body's natural response to trauma and loss is to curl inwards to protect the body's internal organs. In these circumstances, there are more subtle ways to practice backbends.

Where intention goes energy flows—sending breath into your heart can be a more accessible practice until heart openers are available again. This can happen even in forward folds or child's pose by drawing breath in behind your heart. Bringing focus and awareness into this space can be very healing for those craving emotional grounding.

In yoga, heart opening can be a wonderful practice emotionally and spiritually, yet it also has significant physical benefits. Releasing tension around the chest can greatly improve health, especially for anyone with a job that requires them to sit at a desk. More people than ever have careers keeping them seated for prolonged periods of time throughout the day. This sedentary lifestyle can have an impact on posture including shoulder, back, and neck abnormalities which may lead to pain, headaches, and musculoskeletal dysfunction.

Poor posture that results in kyphosis (slumping) from prolonged sitting may contribute to decreased pulmonary function from the effect of gravity impeding the diaphragm. Muscle stiffness through the torso from being sedentary can also lead to restrictive air disease. This makes practicing chest openers more important than ever to counteract these potentially harmful effects. Practicing chest opening regularly will influence heathy posture and breathing.

Louise Hay in her book "You Can Heal Your Life" affirms that all disease comes from a state of unforgiveness—teachings that stem from the work of "A Course in Miracles." What I've noticed working with energy is that certain conditions are derived from specific thoughts or actions.

The idea that we bring on our health issues is eyebrow-raising on the best of days and rage-inducing on others. For anyone who's ever struggled with illness, the thought that we "asked for it" is infuriating. Hear me out: taking responsibility is an act of empowerment. When we open ourselves up to the possibility that our behavior contributes to our healing, it allows us to step back into our personal power.

Even if we only control a small fraction of our health, that fraction puts the power back in our hands. Recovering from or managing a disease is an opportunity to look within our hearts with honesty and integrity to discover what pattern needs to be changed in order to heal.

Typically, this requires forgiveness, a quality that is already an inherent gift of the heart chakra. The body parts that are relevant to this energetic space are the heart, lungs, thymus gland, clavicle, shoulder blades, ribs, arms, hands, and even fingers. The time I ended up with bronchitis highlighted how I could influence my health by healing the patterns I'd adopted.

When I came down with bronchitis, I had just started a 21 day cleansing process through all of the chakras. I knew there was some profound message this experience would give me but it was difficult to see at the time since it felt like I was being punished.

Bronchitis symptoms usually last a couple of weeks—if a case lingers, it could take up to a month. This bout lasted for more than 6 months with some symptoms persisting even after a year. I had trouble sleeping, breathing, and doing regular activities. I was often exhausted from lack of sleep after waking up wheezing in the middle of the night. After numerous trips to an allopathic doctor and alternative health practitioners, I was still determined to get to the root of the issue.

Eventually, one of my teachers introduced me to an amazing osteopath named Warren Hitzig. He sensed an area in my body which was storing my anger. After the appointment, I considered how my thoughts, actions, and emotions contributed to my disease. Looking back on that year, my first thought was that I had been putting my heart and soul into my work as a yoga studio owner. Some of the mundane activities the studio required of me were very time consuming, often leaving me feeling completely drained.

As much as I didn't want to admit it, I realized that I was a limited resource—I couldn't do everything on my own. Not only that, I was bending over backwards for other people instead of saying "no" to the things that either did not resonate or overstepped my personal boundaries. This behavior of people-pleasing created a lot of anger and resentment. Even though I was supporting a space that would allow me to pursue my passions, the act of giving myself away was toxic. It made me less available to do what I really loved, like teaching, while fueling the emotions that created the environment for my disease.

This realization came with many gifts. For one, I looked at my diet to see if it was congruent with what I needed to thrive. I cut out anything that could be related to the inflammation associated with bronchitis symptoms. This change in my habits was a tangible one that supported me on my healing path. The next step was to directly tackle the thoughts and emotions that were holding me back.

One of the toxic thought-patterns I had adopted was that "everything has to be done right now," meaning that any concerns that came up, mostly relating to the studio, had to be addressed immediately. This made every email and request urgent, resulting in a great deal of stress. This caused me to put aside my needs which generated the resentment I had been feeling. A passion of mine that I sacrificed regularly in order to people-please was snowboarding.

Shredding snow is one of the few places outside of yoga and meditation where I can live completely in the moment. It also connected me with my friends which gave me a sense of community outside of the studio. When I realized I needed to change my mindset by putting my needs first, I went through a phase I like to call "fuck it, I'm going snowboarding."

This cheeky phrase meant that I was going to give priority to fun, joy, and presence rather than putting it on the back-burner. It also suggested that most of the items that I thought were "urgent" could wait a few hours to be accomplished. I had to forgive myself for feeling guilty about taking time to do what I truly enjoyed. This allowed me to regain balance in my life which promoted my healing, physically and energetically. My bronchitis, over time and repetition, began to heal.

Another disease I've noticed an energetic link to is breast cancer. Breasts have a strong connection with the heart chakra. They can literally support life by providing nourishment to another human being. Therefore, it makes sense that energetically when we're not careful, we can give too much of ourselves away.

The act of being overly generous—with disregard for the needs of the self—has serious ramifications. Mothers are the most vulnerable to breast cancer due to the mental and emotional patterns that foster this disease. Mothers are under constant pressure to act selflessly by putting the needs of their family and community ahead of their own which creates the energetic conditions for breast cancer to flourish. This pattern of behavior also leaves caregivers and health professionals susceptible as well.

Constantly caring for others while neglecting your own needs has spiritual consequences; without intervention it establishes the perfect storm for disease. Healing requires two mindset shifts: 1.) to forgive yourself when you aren't "perfect." By letting go of this guilt, you give yourself the space to be a human being with needs. These needs—whether they be emotional, intellectual, spiritual, or otherwise—should be met on a regular basis, especially when others depend on you and 2.) putting yourself first is a necessity, not a luxury.

This allows you to fully show up for the people that you love. These perspectives are game-changers on the path to healing. Not only can you support the healing of specific diseases including breast cancer, but you give yourself the freedom to receive for all the work that you do. Knowing that you are worth being cared for, with love, affection, and kindness, will work miracles.

Shifting held beliefs that are oppressing can be a major advantage in fighting disease but the real magic lies in what this new outlook attracts into your life. The heart has an electromagnetic frequency that is much more potent than that of the brain; this frequency is communicating with the rest of the universe.

When it's vibrating at a frequency of love, it is activating the law of attraction. Jack Canfield describes the law of attraction as an effect that is always in motion, working with you even at this very moment. The idea is that what you focus on you will attract; ultimately the outcomes can be positive, negative, or neutral. The universe is responding to the vibrational frequency that you send out through your energy, thoughts, and emotions.

If that has you panicking, here's the good news: every moment is a chance to start again. Each thought or emotion is a seed that you plant. If you tend to that seed with great focus and attention, it will grow. If you notice the seed, and choose not to give it your energy, it will die. Uplifting our energy is as simple as being conscious of the seeds that we plant and what we allow to grow.

Kindness is a seed we must plant often and in abundance. Never underestimate the power of a hug or a gesture of kindness. The arms and hands are an extension of the heart chakra after all, offering us the ability to express love and emotion. This has benefits for the giver and the receiver. As much as kindness can be thought of as thoughtful, caring, and generous, some view it as a form of weakness. This idea that "being kind is for the weak" couldn't be further from the truth.

Kindness reveals an inner strength and vulnerability that radiates out into the world. One small act of kindness has the potential to create a ripple effect, giving kindness and hope to those who may need it most.

If you are ever concerned that someone will take advantage of your kindness, settle back into the strength of the 3rd chakra, Manipura. This will give you the keen guidance and discernment to act compassionately and kindly. Seeing any situation from the other person's perspective, including their background and held beliefs, will allow you to understand the underlying environment that caused their reaction.

Mistaking kindness for always being "rainbows and butterflies" is also a fallacy. Setting firm boundaries is an act of kindness towards yourself. Certain people won't be a fan of when you stand up for yourself and your beliefs, especially if you've played a certain role in their story. For example, I once had a friend who would always ask me for advice but never took it. In fact, she always did the opposite! Eventually, I stopped giving advice which made me feel a lot lighter. Since I played the role of "advice-giver," I risked being labelled unkind, unsupportive, or uncaring. I was lucky that my friend's needs were met by listening without offering up opinions and I no longer had to jump back into that role as the advice-giver. In these situations, being clear about boundaries and acting compassionately is important.

This honours the needs of the other but also sets clear boundaries for your own needs in terms of growth. Be cautious not to let others twist your perception of kindness as we can never control the reactions of other people, only our own response to those reactions.

Never forget that the heart chakra encompasses the ability to heal yourself and others, fueled by love, compassion, and kindness. Although giving ourselves away too much can have negative consequences, we must strive to live a life that shares our heart with others. Just like we can't pour from an empty cup, we must focus on creating space for ourselves first by tapping into our joy and by being willing to practice forgiveness. When we a strike balance by giving to ourselves and performing acts of kindness, we ensure that the heart chakra flourishes.

POSTURES THAT CAN HELP SUPPORT ANAHATA

These are a few postures that support (but are not limited to) the 4th chakra:

- Simple Supported Backbend
- Supported Fish
- Supported Sphinx
- Supported bridge
- Supported heart-opening bridge

12

VISHUDDHA
THE THROAT OR 5TH CHAKRA

When I became a yoga teacher, I was immediately drawn to the spiritual roots of the practice. I knew one day I would go to India to experience yoga from the source. When I signed up for an advanced teacher training intensive in Rishikesh, I felt in my soul it was a time for new beginnings. Although this adventure brought its share of beauty, it also prompted me to face my life with courage—this included reviewing old wounds, unearthing new ones, and navigating new challenges.

My teachers in India offered different perspectives on the practice of yoga which was an eye-opener in many ways. It taught me how I wanted to be defined as a teacher, including which methods did not reflect my values. The knowledge transmitted by my teachers reinforced my love of mantra and meditation but their delivery often felt polarizing.

I did not agree with some of their perspectives on asana practice—aka the postures or physical expression of yoga—and when I asked direct questions regarding asana it was not always clear "why" we practiced them a certain way. It became apparent that tradition was held in high regard, even regularly placed above safety or logical discernment. It was apparent to me that I would have to forge my own path.

However, I was still renegotiating my identity as a yoga teacher. I knew that these new experiences would shape who I was to become but the process left me feeling raw and vulnerable. I was creating a whole new foundation from which to grow from. One experience highlighted this clearly for me.

Near the end of our course we had the opportunity to teach a class for the 200 hour yoga teacher training students. I remember being very nervous while standing in front of this room I was about to lead. Although I'd developed close bonds with some of my 300 hour peers, most of the students that sat before me were complete strangers.

About 5 minutes into teaching the class, I watched a student roll up his mat to promptly leave the room. When he walked out the door I could feel fear taking hold of me. The voice of doubt in my head wouldn't stop repeating the cruel words, "he didn't like your class," and "if only you were a good teacher." I stumbled my way through the rest of the practice with those negative statements lurking in the back of my mind. It didn't help that my teacher sat at the back of the class from beginning to end, shaking his head at me and furrowing his brows in disappointment.

After the class, I remember standing outside on the roof with my teacher, listening to his feedback, like pouring salt in an open wound. Most of his response was a blur but the words that stuck with me were, "you are listening to everyone else. You need to do your own practice."

It was this feedback that briefly shook me awake from my negativity coma. In my head there was a glistening moment that called out, "yes, I do need to do my own practice. I need to share what is in my heart." I knew I could not solely do any other teacher's practice—I had to take the tools given to me and then integrate them in such a way that felt authentic and real, applying them directly to my life and yoga practice—at this point, the "life" and "yoga" didn't seem so separate. This epiphany would be a defining moment that would help me uncover my dharma—or my life purpose.

When I returned back to my room I was still reeling from the embarrassment of having a student leave my class. My mind was churning with the same destructive thought patterns that I couldn't seem to shake. Later that day a group of us gathered outside our yoga school, we planned to check out a café in a different part of town.

While waiting outside I couldn't help but share my insecurities about this mortifying teaching experience. As I relayed the story to this cluster of friends, someone tapped me on the back of the shoulder. When I turned around, the person staring back at me declared, "I was that guy who left your class."

Stunned like a deer in headlights, I stood there with nothing to say—my eyes must have looked like saucers. He continued, "I didn't leave your class because I didn't like it. I left because I thought I was going to shit my pants."

My jaw must have hit the floor. This student leaving class had absolutely nothing to do with me, let alone my teaching. I truly had no idea until he told me that shocking twist! There were two important lessons I learned that day regarding truth:

1. We really have no idea what's happening in someone else's life. Their truth and subsequent reactions reflect their own experiences. This is an excellent reason not to take things personally.

2. Stay connected to your truth—the opinions of others don't define you.

I can think of many other circumstances when this philosophy has served me as a yoga teacher, entrepreneur, and throughout life in general. As a yoga teacher you will always be too fast, too slow, too strong, too soft, too rigid, too creative... for someone out there.

However, when you connect to your truth regardless of how it appears, that energetic presence will attract "the right" people into your life who appreciate an authentic nature.

This applies to attracting the right students as a yoga teacher, romantic partners in relationships, and so much more. Showing up authentically means never having to fit someone else's mold. Just like when you put on an outfit that suits your style—it might not be for everyone, but it fits you perfectly. When authenticity matters more than an outsider's perspective, that outlook provides the freedom to be yourself unapologetically.

Authenticity is an incredible strength of the throat chakra. Without this quality showing up in abundance we are doomed to wander further away from our purpose. The need for power and the path of corruption can drag authenticity right out of the soul, forming a breeding ground for emptiness. This theme shows up regularly in popular culture.

Movies with plots that reveal these dark undertones leave the lead character wildly unhappy—or they appear happy on the surface but unfulfilled on a deeper level—eventually there's an emotional implosion or another method of drastic self-destruction that constitutes the need for a change.

This message is a common theme in reality as well, happening frequently to teens and young adults when they seek belonging and authentic connection from inappropriate sources—excessive drinking, drug abuse, and wild behavior are all symptoms associated with an essential need for belonging. My teenage years and the coping mechanisms I adopted were no exception.

I grew up in a small town where underage drinking was considered "normal." Getting wasted felt fun. It could allow me to be silly, not take anything too seriously, and do what I wanted unapologetically. My friends were in the same boat which helped me fit in socially with little effort. As time went on into my early twenties I began having severe unpredictable reactions to alcohol. Sometimes all it would take was one drink to make me ruthlessly hungover the following day.

This limited me in many ways from living a fulfilled life—it left me in foggy haze constantly with many days spent hanging my head over a toilet. When I hit my mid-twenties I started cutting down on drinking weekly, favouring special events to nights out at a bar—I thought I could triumph over these circumstances. Even when I cut back on my drinking habits, the harsh effects of alcohol on my body persisted.

My body knew the course of action I had to take but my mind resisted. "Can't I just have fun with my friends?" I wondered why I had to be the one who got hungover at the drop of a hat. Embarrassed and frustrated, I ignored the signs that had been thrust upon me, convinced that health tonics and a careful selection of "the right" alcohol could help me get away with drinking.

One year when travelling overseas I met up with an old friend. We drank, laughed, and reminisced. I remember singing and swinging around lamp posts on the way back from the bar. The next day I was heinously hungover. We had to travel by train even though I felt like I could barely move, throwing up multiple times along the journey.

There were many points throughout my teens and into early adulthood when I joked that I was "never drinking again" but something about this day was different. I had finally gotten tired of my own bullshit—I didn't want to waste a single day hungover again. I was ready to take responsibility for this blessing-in-disguise and to finally cut out alcohol once and for all.

It had been clear all this time that alcohol was not meant for me, but it took this long to finally fully accept it. Adjusting to my new lifestyle was surprisingly easy when I started giving less fucks about what other people thought. Those who loved and accepted me embraced the new changes with open arms, those who didn't accept "the new" me pruned themselves out of my life—and they have not been missed. I traded vodka tonics for coconut water and kombucha, I proudly said "no thank you" when someone offered me drinks. I even garnered respect from people I didn't anticipate when I refused drinks. Travelling to Vegas completely sober with my sisters was a blast, I could still be the life of the party without using any substances. I was already fun—dancing, being silly, and enjoying life was completely possible without an alcoholic drink in hand.

The true lesson of this story is in the value of trusting yourself. If you love having drinks with your friends on the weekend, amazing! When your lifestyle choices resonate with your truth, then life flows beautifully. When there are decisions that aren't in alignment with who you are and what you stand for, that's when certain themes appear—and reappear—until you're ready to make the necessary adjustments. My experience in quitting drinking was me finally hitting "rock bottom". Although it wasn't a spectacular disaster by any means, it was the moment I finally felt ready to move on to a new chapter.

As we uncover the parts of ourselves that do not align with the soul, we naturally evolve into who we were always meant to be—freeing ourselves from the circumstances that once dragged us down. With the throat chakra this includes living from a place of truth but also embracing truthfulness through communication. Remaining rooted in kindness and compassion with truthful communication is always within reach even in difficult circumstances. This next story clearly made that lesson quite clear for me.

After I quit drinking I became hyperaware of other people who were under the influence. Although most of my friends were goofy, fun, and in control, there was a dear friend who stood out amongst the rest. I'd always had a hunch that she'd had issues with substances without ever confronting her directly. Gradually as I became more aware of the situation, I realized how deeply this issue ran. When my husband Kevin and I walked down the aisle, she had been drinking heavily and passed out during the speeches at the reception.

My sisters were overwhelmed trying to take care of her, missing many precious moments that would never happen again. When I saw her for the first time after the wedding, I finally faced her regarding how I felt about her drinking. I knew our friendship was on the line at this point even though I cared for her very much and deeply valued our friendship.

Regardless of the love I felt for her, my truth couldn't ignore the fact that this problem was tearing our relationship apart. I could no longer stand idly by and accept this behavior that had caused a great deal of emotional distress time and time again. I voiced my concern for her actions, then explained the clear boundaries for our friendship that had to change—which included no drinking before or during our time together.

It is important to hold space for the people in our life even when they are damaged or going through hardship, however we do not have to withstand destructive behavior. We each have our own truth. Although we can never change someone else, we can honour the expression of our own needs through clear boundaries. If someone's actions are damaging, our responsibility is to either remove ourselves from the situation or communicate clear, compassionate boundaries. In this scenario with my friend, accusations, blame, or guilt were never thrown around needlessly.

When we overcome our own demons it does not give us permission to crucify others for theirs. In these circumstances, moving forward in our friendship demanded clarity delivered in a way that recognized the feelings behind the message—to emphasize that this concern did not stem from judgement, rather it came from a place of love. Just as clear communication is vital to the 5th chakra, doing so in a compassionate way fulfils the qualities of the heart that crave expression. Expressing oneself through the characteristics of each chakra is an inherent part of energetic work.

The throat chakra has a clear theme of expression, highlighting the importance of creativity and communication. This form of communication goes beyond having difficult conversations or conveying our truth, it includes how we speak to ourselves through self-talk.

The inner dialogue of the voice inside our head will be the one who expresses itself the most frequently and it tends to be the loudest. This internal dialogue can quickly turn into an inner critic without careful supervision. Negativity in the form of doubt, self-depreciation, unnecessary complaining, and feelings of worthlessness resonate at a lower frequency than expressions associated with love and gratitude. Everything we communicate about ourselves, whether it is spoken verbally or internally, is heard by our cells—a message the body responds to—and our energetic field—answered by the universe. When we transmit messages about our body in a positive or negative way, the body will match itself to that frequency, responding either positively or negatively.

I've personally noticed this in my yoga practice—my body is always willing to be open and receptive when the internal dialogue is filled with love and appreciation. If my thoughts drift towards criticism, devaluation, and irritation, my body tends to grip, hold, and guard, effectively preventing subtle openings or energetic shifts. We must exercise caution with our thoughts since they create our reality. Even in the darkest places there is room for light, so rather than thinking of the notion as threatening, consider it an opportunity for liberation. How empowering it is to know that every moment and every thought is the chance to plant a new "seed." Seed in this case referring to thought. There were certain people in my life who inspired me to cultivate the best "seeds" possible.

When my dad had cancer he was incredibly strong. While witnessing him as a teenager, I knew he was suffering but I don't remember a single moment he ever complained even as he endured painful chemotherapy treatments, side effects, surgeries, drugs—nothing made him grumble about his condition. Throughout it all there was never a hint of self-pity even when he knew he was dying. He savored the life he had with his limited time on earth and I always deeply respected his tenacity. This quality gave him a beautiful outlook on life leading up to the end, an outlook he would have been robbed of had he focused on the worst of his circumstances. He remained relatively healthy up until his death in part due to the seeds he planted using his positive outlook.

When we nurture these "seeds", that is what we allow to grow in our garden—our garden referring to an overall outlook on life and what that energetic presence attracts. A blossoming garden may pass on more seeds to create more flowers while weeds can have the same impact if they are given the chance. In other words, how we focus our self-talk becomes our reality to attract and repel accordingly. When messages of warmth and love are radiated through inward or outward communication, they will influence how future events unfold. The universe is always listening. The throat chakra thrives on openness, honesty, and creativity, while lies and gossip lead to its decay. This knowledge serves as a warning to be cautious of our words and actions.

At the Obama Foundation Summit, Barack Obama spoke about the poison of judgment and gossip, "if all you're doing is casting stones, you're probably not going to get that far," he affirmed.

This statement holds true for the throat chakra, especially in our response after stones have been thrown in our direction. "Taking the high road" can have so much value for spiritual growth despite how tempting the other path might be. As a yoga teacher and studio owner, there were times when I overheard far-fetched rumours about myself being circulated by other teachers.

As disappointing as this was, I never let it bother me since I knew the universe had a good way of balancing the scales. I chose to move forward with the intention of being my best and brightest self in the process. Years later, I've witnessed the universe respond with all sorts of beautiful seeds flowering in my garden. If I had stayed fixated on those who had wronged me by mirroring their actions, I'd be inviting weeds to grow instead.

The power to attract this beauty and grace was activated by the vibrational frequency of the conscious choice that kept me away from gossip. By choosing to radiate the qualities that served to inspire a life of freedom—from judgement, suppression, and suffering—my energetic field responded to that vibrational frequency in a positive, supportive way.

Every thought, word, and action will transmit a vibrational frequency ranging from low to high— those that are uplifting carry a high frequency while lower frequencies feel draining or diminishing. We are communicating this vibrational frequency that is shared constantly with the universe. The people we come across may also pick up on this frequency which is why someone might pick up on a specific "vibe" that someone radiates. The universe reflects that same vibrational frequency back in the form of opportunities.

The more that high vibrational outputs are exercised to create the life you want, the more those qualities have the potential to show up— love, abundance, peace, joy—all of these states have a vibrational frequency that can be tapped into by communicating the same output. This also translates to words, thoughts, and actions with low vibrational frequencies. When attention is placed on unwanted desires, this is how those negative circumstances can be attracted. Have you ever noticed that the same person voicing their concerns about money never seems to climb out of that rut? No matter what changes in their job or life circumstances their relationship with money never budges. For many, this is tied to mindset. It's very common to unintentionally attract what is constantly being inwardly or outwardly communicated. Just like when my dad had cancer, he chose to focus on the gratitude he had to live out the remainder of his life rather than be pulled down by his circumstances. Gratitude holds an extremely high vibration, working as a powerful super attractor.

Gratitude is known as heart medicine, yet it is also extremely healing for the throat when applied to communication. When life's gifts are recognized and appreciated, it gives more room for abundance to thrive. It's been a regular habit of mine to "thank" the universe for the blessings it has brought. This act doesn't have to be extravagant; it can be as simple as saying "thank you universe for bringing me _____." It does not matter whether this prayer of thanks is said out loud or in thought, transmitting this message clearly and sincerely is what counts. The universe will always pick up on the vibrational frequency sent out in those moments of gratitude, providing new insight that supports us in connecting to our truth.

Sooner or later our truth and dharma reveal themselves to us. Each of us has a different path to travel, just like when my teacher pointed out that I needed to do my own practice. We each have our own "calling" supported by our truth. To follow this unique path authentically is our birthright. No one else can tell us the direction or outcome—and we can't assume someone else's situation either, like when the student left my class unexpectedly.

Our dharma may also have many other pieces of the puzzle that support us along the way. When I quit drinking, this shift created a lot more space than I ever thought possible, granting me a more fulfilled life. Part of this fulfillment was enabled through the throat chakra by enforcing firm yet compassionate boundaries as well as avoiding the downfalls of judgement and gossip. Committing to decisions from this place of warmth always serves our thoughts, words, and actions—in turn, creating the reality that unfolds. Finally, applying gratitude as the "cherry on top" supports calling in any gifts we seek—by communicating gratitude we become empowered to attract miracles.

POSTURES THAT CAN HELP SUPPORT VISHUDDHA

These are a few postures that support (but are not limited to) the 5th chakra:

- Legs Up the Wall (with bolster under hips)
- Supported Bridge
- Supported Heart Opening Bridge

13

AJNA

THE THIRD EYE OR 6TH CHAKRA

In spring of 2019 my husband, Kevin, and I launched an organic, plant-based food truck. During the time leading up to our opening weekend, we were seeking suppliers to provide everything from recipe ingredients to to-go containers. We wanted to choose suppliers that were in alignment with our values, knowing that one of our highest priorities was to find environmentally conscious options.

We were out for lunch one day when Kevin caught the eye of a woman sitting at a nearby table. He walked up to her almost immediately to say, "do I know you?" I stood there, watching their interaction. Looking at this woman, I had a feeling he did not know her. I felt like I was witnessing an awkward conversation unfold as they were going back and forth trying to figure where they could know each other from.

The woman radiated warmth and patience during this interaction, even though I could tell she had no idea who he was. When Kevin asked where she worked, she mentioned that she'd left her recent job to spread the word about edible straws. Edible straws?! We had no idea such a product existed. Before that moment we'd found some compostable straws which were "ok" for our food truck but this product was better than anything we'd come across. Having this option for the beverages we were offering was a perfect fit! We exchanged contacts so that we could purchase these straws for our new business.

When we left the café, I turned to Kevin and asked, "What made you want to talk to her?" I was amazed he'd stumbled upon this invention that was instrumental to our new business. He told me he felt compelled to talk to this person—this "pull" would override his sense of fear, insecurity, and potential embarrassment. In fact, he didn't even think of the consequences. Kevin was acting on pure instinct, a deeper knowledge that he couldn't explain. Deep down he knew he couldn't leave without introducing himself.

Kevin's strong intuition is a perfect example of the power of the 6th chakra, Ajna. This is our center of wisdom, intuition, and knowledge. This sense of "knowing" goes beyond our basic understanding of the world. For anyone who's ever walked into a space to feel the "vibe" of a room, there's a clear presence that feeds back to our intuitive nature. We have the capacity to feel what events may have happened there or the type of person that has occupied the space, perhaps even the emotions they've expressed. It's like an imprint in the air that lingers long after a person is gone.

Even science backs this idea of being able to pick up on good or bad "vibes." De Groot et al, a team of Dutch researchers, showed that humans could detect chemosignals by smelling bodily excretions— like sweat or tears—left over from people who had been in that location. In this study they had one group wear a specific t-shirt while watching either a scary or disgusting video. These shirts were then given to a different group who were asked to smell them. Those who received the "fear sweat" shirts reacted with a fearful expression while those who had "disgust sweat" had a disgusted expression.

A follow-up study discovered that positive emotions could be transmitted in the same way. For anyone who's ever picked up on bad vibes from a person or a place, this research just confirms what we already knew: these signals are palpable. I'd even go a step further to say that spiritual residue from our energetic field (aka our aura) can linger in the spaces we occupy. Our presence can extend beyond our physical body, and just like our sweat or tears that can be left behind or sensed by other people, so can our energy signature.

There may be situations in which your intuition begs you to take a step forward or a step back based on these "vibes." You might even feel that you instantly "know" someone and what a good person they are even after you just met them. Perhaps this is how I had such a positive experience in this next story.

While visiting India, I was out browsing the shops one day when I found the perfect gift for a close friend of mine: a unique handmade journal. There weren't many left and without enough money to purchase it, I was worried I'd be out of luck by coming back another day. I was chatting with the shopkeeper and while flipping through the pages he asked me if I wanted to buy it.

When I told him my situation and that I'd have to come back, he told me "it's fine, take it. You can pay me tomorrow." I was floored. Pay him tomorrow? How does he know that I'm not just going to take it without ever paying him? I was a foreigner he'd never met before! The amount of trust he had was shocking and heart-warming. I thought about how this would never happen back home with someone who didn't know me, especially with a more expensive purchase like this one. I thanked him and planned to pay him the next day.

When I arrived back where I was staying, I realized that I couldn't get back to the shop until the day after. Seeing the shopkeeper two days later, I apologized profusely for being a day late but his reaction was calm and kind. He didn't have a doubt in his mind about me coming back to settle the tab. Intuitively, he knew that I would honour my debt. He held an understanding of my character without "knowing" me, through a deep level of faith in his intuition. The kindness, warmth, and trust he exuded inspired me. It acted as a reminder that sometimes we need to put ourselves out there, even at the risk of being burned, when our intuition gives us the green light. By having this trust, we honour our intuition and put our faith back into humanity. We can learn to decode these signals by picking up on the "vibes" of those around us.

Author and speaker Caroline Myss sums it up perfectly, "your intuition automatically reads the energy of everyone around you. Every living being is made up of energy and all of this energy contains information. Your physical body is surrounded by an energy field that is both an information clearing center and a highly sensitive perceptual system. We are constantly communicating with everything around us, with the greater energy of the universe and the consciousness of other living creatures. Our energy field sends and receives messages to and from other people and these internal and external messages form energy impressions that are picked up by our intuition."

The explanation provided by Caroline thoroughly describes intuition. We are constantly sending and receiving information that reacts with our environment. The signals that we radiate outwards depend on our thoughts, emotions, and current state, which each leave energetic impressions. Information that is perceived comes through "translators" also known as the chakras. Although our 6th chakra is the center of intuition, there is a clear relationship with intuition and the other energy centers involved in our spiritual development.

If you've ever felt the need to "trust your gut" about a decision, then you understand the internal reaction related to the 3rd chakra. The same principle applies to the idea behind "following your heart." In other words, each energetic center plays a role in responding to the environment, supported by the knowledge of the 6th chakra.

Fear is a common barrier to the development of intuition. Innate wisdom is not a difficult skill to cultivate when fear stands aside. The major hurdle when nurturing this gift is to clearly see the difference between fear and intuition. Discernment between the two happens with the contribution of truth and honesty from the throat chakra. In situations where fear could be confused with intuition, digging deeper to see the truth creates useful insight. Examples of the confusion between fear and intuition come from my experiences in hiring teachers at the studio.

A teacher I already knew approached me about a teaching position at the studio. We both had taught at a different location in our community so we had been acquainted with one another for nearly a year. I asked her to submit an application, then we could get together so she could demonstrate her teaching style to me as I hadn't attended her classes.

One of the requirements that's mentioned in our application asks that our teachers provide their teaching insurance. I firmly believe all teachers should have an active policy when offering public classes, just in case, to protect oneself in unforeseen circumstances. This agreement would defend a teacher in a worst-case scenario so it's something that I take seriously. When this teacher applied, I remember there were negative comments made about having to get teaching insurance. I was surprised this was something she didn't have already, especially since she was actively teaching public classes. When I explained that this was more for her than it was for me, she begrudgingly conceded. This was my first red flag. My intuition was already on high alert but I neglected those hints on this first bump in the road of our professional relationship.

When we met for our demo, I remember working through her class to find other red flags pop up, signaling that she may not be a good fit for the studio. Despite these warnings, I went against what I could feel in favour of hiring her. My "logical" brain overpowered all of the intuitive hunches I had been feeling. This voice of practicality told me she was an experienced teacher, not to mention the fact that I'd known her previously gave me a false sense of security.

Over the coming months I remember having a few comments about her classes, even a few complaints. When I addressed a deeply concerning allegation with her, she had a very strong reaction. I gave her an explanation as to what behaviors weren't working but it wasn't clear whether she was truly open to receiving the feedback. Despite this doubt, I still let things slide. I had only been a studio owner for a couple of years, this was my first time dealing with a situation like this. I hadn't fully stepped into my power as a leader to make decisions that benefitted the whole studio community, which included aligning with the right teachers.

This made me feel conflicted as I also wanted to have compassion for this person, but in hindsight, the most compassionate action would've been to set boundaries right away. When I finally let this teacher go, it was a disheartening experience for all involved. Looking back, there were many moments when my intuition tried to advise me but I pushed it out in favour of what was practical or polite. Fear can often mask itself as practicality, politeness, or responsibility. These characteristics were not congruent with my truth or my intuition, which is likely why it blew up in my face. Under other circumstances, the scenario may have been very different.

For instance, I have had similar confrontations with other teachers but did not have the same feedback from my intuition. In some cases, there may be a probable reason for fear but an intuitive compass offers up a different perspective, just like in this next story.

A teacher who had taught with us for about a year decided it was time to start her own studio. Knowing how much heart and soul goes into a project like that, I wished her well in her endeavor. A number of our teachers ended up joining her staff—some studio owners may be shaken by this but I am a firm believer that every space has a unique concept, intention, and energy to hold space for.

Students would naturally be drawn to the community that provided the right fit for them—just as a student is drawn to certain teachers, the same concept applies to choosing a studio. Eventually, the new studio closed. After a few months, she reached out to me to see if she could rejoin our teaching staff. When I looked deep within my intuition, no alarm bells went off—there were zero signals telling me to be cautious of deception. On the surface, it'd be easy to assume otherwise but my intuition was very clear that I could trust this person. I rehired this teacher and although she is no longer leading classes in the studio, we parted ways on very good terms. I was reaffirmed that this decision had a positive outcome by listening to my intuitive resources.

In very similar circumstances, I have made different conclusions based on the pull of my inner guide. This highlights the significance of seeing each scenario from a fresh lens, one that stems from truth and acts upon the assistance of our intuition. This ability to integrate truth into the equation blossoms from the strength of the energy in the throat. The impact of the 5th chakra influences the potential of the 3rd eye—or ajna—emphasizing the importance of building upon each chakra sequentially.

Each "step" starting with the 1st chakra supports the next energetic center, rather than attempting to work backwards from the crown. Each chakra has its strengths which will only be bolstered by the power of the chakras beneath it. Imagine your energetic systems are like building a pyramid, the foundation must be strong and secure rather than being smaller or less supportive than those that sit above. Although the higher chakras are essential for our spiritual development, we need to have a strong foundation to grow from.

One of the attributes associated with spiritual growth is empathy—a quality the world needs now more than ever. Empathy asks us to reach out with our hearts by placing ourselves in someone else's shoes so we can develop an understanding of that individual's actions, emotions, or circumstances. This sense of compassion gives us a clear view of the world to recognize the connections we share with others on an emotional level.

The concept of being an "empath" takes this notion a step further. Judith Orloff, M.D. explains that being an empath is about having empathy, but on a completely different level. She also states that empaths not only feel for others, but they absorb those feelings in their own system. This is how the chakras process that intuitive information. Those who are empaths can pick up on subtle unspoken feelings or the information from someone's energetic field which are key strengths of the 6th chakra. Sometimes this can feel like a curse but those who have this ability are truly blessed when that power is used wisely, just like in this next encounter.

While teaching a restorative class, I offered a beloved student a hands-on adjustment. I knew she was going through a rough time in her life due to a recent break-up from her partner. I was adjusting the area around her pelvis, an energetic space that tends to be associated with relationships and emotional energy, when I felt overwhelming sadness wash over me. It was so intense I thought I might burst into tears. I could feel the depth of her sadness nestled into her energetic field.

I fully experienced her suffering and in that instant of vulnerability there was no judgement—her emotions were not "good" or "bad"—I could only radiate warmth and love towards her. To show up in this way for other people is the best way to create a safe container for them to express themselves. This ability is known as "holding space," a common process adopted naturally by most empaths, caregivers, or light workers. During this act of holding space, the concentration of the emotion I experienced was a perfect example of how empaths integrate these energy transfers.

Despite having these types of experiences for some time now, I never considered myself an empath until more recently. My justification being that I tend not to "take on" other people's energy which is commonly associated being an empath. What I've come to realize is that it's possible to develop this gift without processing or storing other people's spiritual "junk." For those who are energetically sensitive this should be a relief. Just as you can be around a person with a cold or flu and never get sick, there are ways to defend against certain spiritual illnesses as well. There are a few ways to repel darker, heavier forms of energy, and with practice they are easy habits to adopt.

The first is to prioritize setting clear and appropriate boundaries. Examples of setting boundaries would be saying "no" in certain circumstances, specifically in situations that are physically, mentally, or emotionally draining. Another example would be limiting interactions with people that you know will "bring you down" energetically. If that's not possible, focus on being a beacon of light. A flashlight can brighten up even the darkest spaces. In those moments when we are being "tested," focus on being that bright light with emotions, language, and presence. Above all, it is our responsibility to maintain compassion for the human being that is stuck in that darkness, even if that means creating space from that person.

A technique for protection that many energetic practitioners use, including myself, involves visualization. This is especially helpful for those who respond well to visual stimuli either for learning or focus. In this visualization, envision yourself covered in white light, one that makes you feel held and supported. Continue to imagine this white light that does not allow anything to penetrate it—this space you hold for yourself only allows positivity and light to enter. If you feel you need an extra "layer", then create an additional protective shield of mirrors around the light, allowing outside energy to be reflected away.

The best piece of guidance I can offer when it comes to holding space for others is this: each of us energetically allows people and situations into our lives. Perhaps these circumstances are meant to elevate, teach, and cultivate wisdom regardless of whether the experience seems positive or negative. In these social interactions—when intuition often comes in handy—we are all doing the best we can with what we have. There are people out there who may have less "tools" in their spiritual toolbox to draw from, yet we must hold space for them all the same. Controlling another's perception is like trying to guide a kite in an unpredictable hurricane, it's impossible! We can only meet them as deeply as they have met themselves.

Your intuition is meant to assist you in navigating these relationships to discover how to hold space for you and for the people you come across. Rather than always defaulting to a logical checklist for answers, it is our duty to "see" and "feel" without using our typical senses. The outcomes that emerge from using intuition can be used to fully understand the true connections that we share energetically with the world.

PRACTICES THAT CAN HELP SUPPORT AJNA

These are a few techniques that support (but are not limited to) the 6th chakra:

- Meditation
- Brahmari
- Nadi shodana (best with first two fingers resting on 3rd eye)
- Bringing internal gaze to the 3rd eye (while meditating or while eyes are closed in a posture)

14

SAHASRARA
THE CROWN OR 7TH CHAKRA

When I was participating in a teacher training in India, I had an awakening on one of the first evenings during meditation. My teacher had left the room, leaving me and my peers sitting still for quite some time. I started to feel my energy shift to the point where I could see my breath linked to a glowing light that expanded and contracted for every inhale and exhale. Afterwards it became clear this was my aura —the electromagnetic field that radiates out from every living being.

When my teacher returned, I could see their aura even with my eyes closed. As time passed, I saw shapes moving, coiling, unfurling, and sparkling in the darkness with an overwhelming sense of bliss settling in. Suddenly my mind went, "this must be enlightenment!" The minute that my conscious mind identified this experience, "poof" it was gone. When the meditation was over, I felt like I had been drugged. I left the room in a joyful yet calm daze which permeated into the hours that followed. I couldn't quite figure out what I'd stumbled upon but I knew that it was a step in my spiritual development.

After that night, I yearned for those feelings to return—I was determined to reach this enlightened state. If I had done it once, surely I could do it again. I showed up night after night for meditation expecting this bliss to return—after all, I had already felt this intense download of divine consciousness—but it was always just out of reach. Shortly after that evening, a different teacher began teaching mantra during meditation, which made me feel even more frustrated. "Why are we singing mantra when we should be still?" I thought, stewing away and rolling my eyes.

I felt I was being pulled from my "goal." The more that I lusted to relive those moments, the further away it seemed. This is the struggle a lot of practitioners have with the 7th chakra, Sahasrara. When a taste of divinity and grace is given, immediately there is an expectation for that pinnacle to be repeated with ease. Although it's not impossible, there is no guarantee. In fact, being "blocked" from that experience can be a spiritual test itself. This test urges practitioners to ask themselves: can you continue your yoga and meditation practice without the need to achieve enlightened states? For many, this is like the carrot dangling just out of reach. Most practitioners will continue to chase, seeing this as the goal rather than appreciating it as a "bonus." Any person who sets foot on the spiritual path needs to be aware of this trick.

Fortunately, you don't have to fall into this trap. There are so many gifts that the 7th chakra brings—divine connection, sense of belonging, and an understanding of the light—serving as a gatekeeper for creation, love, and healing. Light in this sense is a relationship with source, describing what some refer to as "god" or universal energy. Yoga, reiki, or any form of energy healing is not a requirement to form a connection with source.

In fact, there are many ways to nurture this relationship. Some may discover this union through yoga and meditation while others feel a higher power through mantra and prayer. Light energy, universal life force, and god can offer these gifts to anyone who is open to receiving them. The 7th chakra is all about opening yourself up to this divine light to realize your place in the world through your relationship with the entire universe.

A wise mentor once told me that anyone could connect to light, even those who don't feel they are spiritual can be touched by grace. Although I agree with this sentiment, it can separate vulnerable people from their spiritual potential. This statement is like saying, "just eat healthy" to someone who's eaten junk food their entire life. To transition that quickly without a clear-method of practice or repetition does not work well long-term, leaving those without this foundation back in their same habitual patterns with no safety net. Just like the junk food addict being told to "eat healthy" without any guidance, the spiritual seeker will end up doubting their faith and themselves.

When I've taught others about energy, the 7th chakra is often the least understood of the energetic centers. It is not something that can be taught or experienced directly. To know this chakra, it must be felt on a soul level. To feel divine connection means there is a deep trust that our life and what occurs in it, good and bad, lines up with our purpose —in the sense that the universe is always working with us rather than against us. It also recognizes each person as a spiritual being having a human experience instead of the other way around.

There are many moments that can make us forget this divine wisdom. That's also the beauty of having a human experience; we are designed to be flawed and to make mistakes. This is part of how we self-actualize. Can you imagine if we were always perfect and never made mistakes? How easy life would be! Would you have the same level of compassion, appreciation, understanding, and wisdom? Life is meant to have obstacles which help us grow. This is part of our divine purpose—even when it makes you roll your eyes and sigh.

Spiritual experiences can be brought about with plant medicines or drugs; this can be a very valuable experience to hold space for healing. I do caution those who tend to lean on this method since spiritual wisdom comes from within—not through substances, people, or things. When it comes to fostering a closer connection to universal consciousness, drugs will show you the door but they won't give you the key. Only you have the key. There is no teacher, drug, book, podcast, or any other tangible thing that can open that door for you. Knowledge and understanding through these resources are beautiful tools but without the acknowledgement that each of us is responsible for our own spiritual awakening, we are lost.

The spiritual evolution that is happening in this era makes it a fascinating time to be alive. At a point where more people are evolving to wake up to their true potential, we are also dealing with a deep level of darkness and despair. These events are no coincidence. With the opening of the higher chakras, new challenges are brought forth to assist us in the process of self-actualization. Although these events may feel unsettling or even jarring at times, this process is meant to assist us in learning and growing as we navigate our time on earth.

Brené Brown has a refreshing outlook on nourishing our spiritual needs. She says, "Spirituality is recognizing and celebrating that we are all inextricably connected to each other by a power greater than all of us, and that our connection to that power and to one another is grounded in love and compassion. Practicing spirituality brings a sense of perspective, meaning and purpose to our lives."

The power of the 7th chakra resides in an understanding of our connection with the rest of the universe. That our "being" has a direct line with the people who cross our path, our experiences, and that our purpose plays a greater role in the bigger picture than just what lies in our immediate future. I've always found it so fascinating that meditation stimulates our sense of grounding, identity, and feelings of being at "home" related to the 1st chakra, yet the connection to the 7th chakra is also so clear. There are many reasons for this, but one explanation stands out: the key to who we really are is inextricably linked to source. When we are steady and stable in ourselves, it naturally illuminates the pathway to divine consciousness.

Phrases like "divine consciousness" and "universal source energy" can seem unrealistic or unreachable if you feel out of the spiritual loop but these states of bliss are available to everyone. Connecting to this potential is simple—it's the ability to see grace every day, in the mundane, and even in the grit. Appreciating the beauty in its humblest forms. Standing on top of a mountain looking across a vast landscape or looking into the eyes of a child. Anytime that you feel effortless gratitude and joy for this gift of life you've been given.

These don't just happen in the happy, joyous moments. In fact, the most powerful shifts can happen when beauty is seen in darker times, because "god" in all its affirmations lives in the grit beneath your fingernails. One of my teachers, Ana Forrest, said to take the shit into your life and turn it into fertilizer. This is exactly what god, infinite consciousness, or divine purpose wants you to do. Rather than be stifled and broken, this energetic force wants you to bloom like the lotus flower rising from the grimiest muck at the bottom of the pond. The events in your life are not happening to you, they are happening for you. Understanding this concept will guide you, but feeling it in your soul is a way of liberating yourself from suffering.

The universe is always working with you rather than against you. Even in the darkest moments, it is trying to guide you in the right direction. Our energy, thoughts, and emotions are always in communication with this divine power—it is always ready to respond right back to us. In an interview with Louise Hay, she discussed the power of affirmations as well as the principle of believing that only good can come to you. She said that when a client comes to her saying a prosperity affirmation hasn't worked, she would ask them, "how many poverty affirmations did you do?" Perhaps they did three prosperity affirmations, but throughout the day they included three-hundred detrimental affirmations.

Words like "I can never get ahead" or "I am not good enough" attract more of those circumstances. Internal dialogue influences what we attract depending on what runs through our mind from sun-up to sun-down. The universe is always there to provide us with everything we need if we are ready to receive it. Manifesting is a perfect example of the gifts that can be provided when we align ourselves with that reality. What we project into the world through our thoughts and actions is what guides us into that alignment. The circumstances of this next situation led me to believe the universe had my back.

One morning I was getting ready to head out the door when I noticed there was a run in my tights. I thought to myself "oh well, I guess I better start looking for new ones." Later that day I noticed an email in my personal inbox from a business that I did not recognize. Rather than disregard it as spam, I went with my intuition to open it. It was from a company that created "unbreakable" tights that boasted that they're 10x stronger than steel. Not only was it from a company that could provide me with exactly what I needed, the email was asking if I would like to be gifted a pair of their tights of my choice! I couldn't believe my luck. I hadn't heard of the company before—I didn't even know such an amazing product existed—and the email was directly to my inbox rather than through the studio. I wasn't even sure how she had been able to reach out to me directly and address me by name.

At the time, I did not have a big online presence or contacts in all-the-right places. All I knew is that this was a blessing. This confirmed that the universe was listening and replying by working its magic through the woman who reached out to me through email. This small act reaffirmed to me that when we are open and ready to receive, it's possible to experience these little miracles. Sometimes, much quicker than expected!

Another experience I had helped me write this book. In spring of 2019 I was leading a restorative yoga teacher training. I'd been offering this type of training for a few years at this point using a book resource from a teacher I highly respected. Even though I agreed with most of the information, this text was far from my "ideal" learning material to supplement the program.

Before our morning session, about halfway through the program, I went up the mountain for a few laps on my snowboard. I was sitting on a chairlift, reflecting on the incongruences between my teaching and the book resource I was using when I had an epiphany: I had to write a book. I had known for years that I wanted to write a book, I just wasn't sure what the content or focus would be. In this moment I knew exactly how my knowledge and expertise would serve the world. It was like some divine presence bopped me on the head that day while cruising through the clouds on that chairlift to say "wake up! This is what you need to do."

When the afternoon session started, I was showing students a photo in the book resource we were using to explain how and why I would do this posture differently. One of the students spoke up to say, "You need to write a book!" When I looked around, all the students were nodding their heads in agreeance. Well, that did it. Not only did divine energy download some inspiration, it reaffirmed through my students that very same day! I knew that I would be supported in getting this project done, but I still wasn't completely sure how. I remember writing the beginning of this book, lacking direction, knowledge, and insight, but trusting that somehow I would figure it out along the way.

Flash-forward another month—I am at a café in a neighboring town with my husband. On one of the walls, there's a large bulletin board with a million messages on it. The whole board is filled to the brim with information—thousands of words, promotional material, and contacts splattered on the wall from business cards to posters. I don't usually pause to look at these but when I came out of the washroom, my eyesight zeroed in on one small message: "Want to write your book?" I was stunned. This was exactly what I was looking for!

There it sat, on a large sheet, in tiny letters, next to multiple other taglines. It was no bigger than two of the lines in this book. I couldn't believe my luck or divine timing! This is exactly what I had been asking for, delivered in the most subtle way. I took a photo of the information so I could reach out that very same day. This is how I met my book coach, Mike Skyrpnek. I knew throughout this process that I had been supported every step of the way. This story is another beautiful example of how an idea, thought, or emotion can manifest into reality.

Rather than thinking of manifesting as "spiritual Santa Claus," consider it a way of aligning yourself with opportunity. Journaling and vision boards will never materialize if the inner work is avoided—the energetic presence needs to match the aspirations. Our beliefs and behaviours hold energy. When that energy meets what we are seeking, those possibilities reveal themselves to us. Faith is the final piece of that puzzle, to know that we are supported in all that we do. When we surrender and trust that the universe has our back, space is created for miracles. The universe has its own plan for us, we just need to pay attention to the signs that come our way so we can shine like we are all meant to.

Sometimes we forget our spiritual nature. Anger, frustration, or sadness can pull us away from our divine self—these mindsets may even attract experiences that limit spiritual freedom. Although all emotions hold value, it is up to us to uncover what is helpful and what is harmful in any given situation. When you feel these expressions are blocking you from your true spiritual nature, the best defense is to catch yourself in those instances when your attention wanders to negativity, then consciously choose to come back to your true self.

Some situations are harder to catch while some days it will take longer than expected—especially if you are physically, mentally, or emotionally exhausted—but it's never too late to start getting "good" at catching yourself in those moments. When you get skilled at "catching" yourself, you are rewiring your brain to use those neural pathways again in the future. Soon, unnecessary negativity will get bypassed since your thoughts have been pre-programmed for positivity.

Even positive experiences may seem like they draw attention away from our spirit but this is actually part of the journey. If we were always in a state of seriousness, contemplating the universe with all of its eccentricities, we would never have the opportunity to experience what it means to be human. This humanness stems from our ability to make mistakes and to be in a process of learning which develops humility. Humour is a beautiful way to cultivate humility. Laughter and childlike play, in Sanskrit known as "lila," is a divine expression that can lead to spiritual growth.

One of my favourite stories that illustrates this perfectly comes from Hindu mythology about Krishna as a child. In this tale, young Krishna and his brother Balaram were playing in the courtyard when Krisha decided to take a scoop of earth in his hands and eat it. Balaram ran to tell their mother, Yashoda, what had happened. Their mother angrily confronted Krishna, eventually demanding that he open his mouth.

When he finally conceded, she did not find any dirt or mud in his mouth, rather she saw the whole universe and all of its galaxies. Although Krishna's parents and friends knew of his divinity, his childlike nature made them forget. This form of lila facilitates the highest type of connection that the soul can have to universal spirit. The forgetfulness they experienced allowed Krishna's family to play, joke, and laugh with him in a way that would not be possible if they were fully conscious of his divinity. It is this forgetfulness that allows us to stay engaged with the world in a meaningful way while staying connected to our soul.

Caroline Myss in her book "Invisible Acts of Power" mentions another story from Hindu legend that hints at our divine connection. In this fable, all human beings were gods but they lacked appreciation for their power, leading the other gods to take it from them. Brahma, the supreme god, sought to hide divinity in a place that humans would never find it. One god suggested that it be placed deep inside the earth. Brahma concluded that humans would eventually dig it up. Another god thought they should set it on the highest mountain. Brahma determined that humans would one day climb it. This frustrated the council of the gods since they knew that sooner or later humans had the potential to conquer any place on earth. Finally, Brahma realized that if they were to hide their divinity within their own being, humans would never think to look for it there. We have been seeking our divinity ever since.

Although pursuing happiness through experiences like travelling or education can be enriching, these encounters alone will never elevate the spiritual self. It is up to each of us to navigate our inner world in order to fully understand our divine presence. Connecting with and remembering our own divine nature is not meant to be difficult, it is our birthright! We have this divine consciousness outside and within ourselves to reveal. When we release the gunk that does not resonate with our soul, the true self is revealed effortlessly. Staying on "the path" requires us to identify our true place in the universe, including the signs it brings, while staying true to ourselves in a playful and forgiving way.

RESTORATIVE POSTURES THAT CONNECT TO THE 7TH CHAKRA

The postures in restorative yoga that connect us with the 7th chakra are those that bring us closer to light, "god," or infinite consciousness. They remind us of our true nature when so many things in the world make us forget. That mission is to live in a state of love, which is what this energy is all about. Although all restorative postures create a state of relaxation and ease that can bring us into that "flow," there are only two shapes meant to have that direct intention: savasana and meditation. Other postures may connect to the crown when we invite the qualities of meditation into the practice.

15

RESTORATIVE POSTURES

SAVASANA AKA CORPSE POSE

We are in a constant state of change from birth to death and there's no reason to hang onto the parts of ourselves that have been outgrown. The idea of practicing "corpse pose" is meant to be reassuring. Yes, this posture is about death. Death of the previous self, old or stagnant ideas, and the person who you once were. Some find this concept terrifying, yet this process is intended to be liberating! Letting go of the dead parts of ourselves that no longer fit gives the butterfly an opportunity to emerge from the chrysalis. Transformation leads to freedom.

Savasana is the chance to renew ourselves every single time we practice it. Naturally, it usually comes at the end of the practice, but it can also be used as a transition between postures as a form of integration or as a way of grounding at the beginning of your sequence. Just like life, the cycles of birth, life, death, and rebirth don't just occur once, they happen constantly. New beginnings are transpiring in every moment. Practicing savasana is a way of trusting the process that's unfolding while opening the self up to new and exciting possibilities.

How long?

Savasana is an essential posture—it should be incorporated into every practice, even if just for a short period of time. For an hour-long practice 10 minutes is recommended while 15 minutes would be ideal for 1 hour and 15 minutes. Including savasana at the end of the practice is perfect to support the full integration of the entire practice within the nervous system and energetic field. Just as sleep is essential for our physical health, our time on the mat requires rest to support the new neurological pathways that have been made. For our energetic well-being, the act of shedding and renewal as we shift into alternate brain states allows those pathways to make positive connections, creating the potential for major shifts mentally and emotionally.

What Props

Savasana is the only posture that does not require specific props, there is only suggested support depending on what you feel you need to be truly relaxed. If the ground is comfortable, with adequate space, this posture can be practiced nearly anywhere, preferably using an even, hard surface to lie on—a mat may also be useful. Choosing a hard surface is preferable because it helps to realign the spine.

This is better done on a hard surface than on a soft bed or couch due to Newton's 3rd Law: every action has an equal and opposite reaction. In this case, the first action is the weight of gravity. Meaning, the ground pressing up into the body has a more significant impact that results in these structural changes. Just like if you were to apply pressure to a solid block between your thighs—rather than a pillow—the block would create more resistance. Another principle known as specific adaptation to implied demand—aka the SAID principle—supports this theory suggesting that with the assistance of gravity a harder surface can realign the spine into its natural state and can even correct minor spinal malformations.

The only case in which a hard surface would not be ideal is when a person has a health concern related to the spine that causes pain when pressure is applied. There are numerous conditions that can cause discomfort when lying down flat which can be adapted for by using additional props or practicing a different shape with a similar intention.

Suggested / Optional props:

Bolster

- underneath knees
- avoid placing underneath back unless there is a condition to support

Blanket

- mild blanket roll underneath neck—just enough to support the curve of the cervical spine (i.e. vertebrae in neck) with excess blanket lightly folded underneath the back of head
- can be used overtop body for warmth
- useful for mild spinal conditions that may require additional cushion

Some students create a large pillow to prop up their head. Although this seems tempting, it creates flexion in the cervical spine—the spine in your neck—which means it's not in a neutral position. Ideally, your spine has its natural curvatures so only a light support under the head is encouraged

Eye pillow

- over closed eyelids
- an eye pillow resting on each hand, in the palm (palms facing up)

Sandbag

- Overtop pelvis resting overtop from hip bone to hip bone
- One on each leg or one on each arm

Is there any substitute for Savasana?

The short answer is, no. Savasana has a specific intention regarding the energetic applications for any yoga practice. There is no additional stretch or release intended in the posture besides coming back to neutral. This is the only posture that offers "no" pose, and for good reason.

The express purpose is to "do" nothing; and doing nothing cannot be substituted. The relaxation of tissues in this position offers no release other than what occurs mentally, emotionally, and spiritually. Essentially this pose acts as our "reset" button with the bonus of holding space for us to leave the heavy baggage behind. This has a physical benefit as well since the nervous system is able to integrate the positive neurological connections that have been made.

This ensures healthy neural networks that are hardwired for relaxation in the future. Other reclined postures—Baddha Konasana (butterfly) or Viparita Karani (legs up the wall)—have a different focus energetically and offer gentle openings in the tissues. Despite being wonderful shapes to practice they do not replicate the effects offered by Savasana as the ultimate neutral rest. While other postures can also be grounding, calming and restful, there is no substitute for a true death of the practice.

Exceptions to this rule:

A variation is recommended when there is pain while practicing a traditional savasana. Under these circumstances, taking a relaxing position with the absence of pain would be more beneficial to fully absorb the benefits of the practice. This could be lying on your side, resting on a bed, or even in a comfortable chair. Location is less important than mindset and the presence you call in as you practice this shape

After the 1st trimester of pregnancy lying on the left side is recommended. This is to keep the vena cava vein free and open. When the fetus grows there is a reorganization of internal organs and blood vessels, putting additional pressure on the inferior vena cava, a major vein that carries deoxygenated blood away from the heart. The compression of the inferior vena cava can mean less blood flow back to the heart which may lead to an unhealthy drop in blood pressure for both mom and baby, resulting in a decrease in the flow of oxygen.

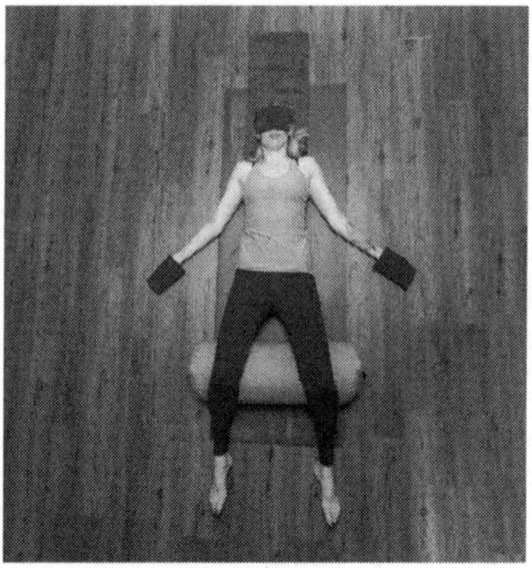

Fig. 15.1

How To

How each person chooses to practice savasana depends solely on what feels comfortable. Each of the following alignment instructions is a suggestion rather than a definitive approach.

- Feel can be wide, even mat distance apart. Don't feel afraid to take up space
- Tailbone lengthens towards feet, giving your lower back more space

- Shoulders release away from ears and sink into the earth
- Arms are heavy, palms are open skywards

Although palms down can be beneficial in some circumstances like in meditation, it can be too stimulating for the sensory receptors in the hands during savasana.

Palms facing up is also a gesture to receive energy from the universe. Energetically, it signals "I am ready to receive" indicating openness and can be useful for increasing manifesting potential

- Back of your neck is long and throat is relaxed
- Back of head is heavy
- Soften muscles of face, including forehead, space between brows, and jaw
- Let go of any breath techniques—invite your breath to soften and smooth. Breath naturally without any effort.

Suggestions for Coming Out of the Posture

- bring movement to fingers and toes, then ankles and wrists
- turn head side to side
- take a long, deep stretch with arms and legs whilst inhaling deeply, release with exhale
- draw knees into chest, give a gentle squeeze, rock side to side or make circles with knees (both directions)
- rest to one side. Traditionally, the right side is associated energetically with the more masculine, intense, fiery energy like the sun—rolling to this side is more appropriate in the morning and early afternoon. The left side is related to the feminine, nurturing, softer energy like the moon which is perfect for later in the day into the evening.

You can rest your head on your mat or use your arm as a pillow, whatever feels more comfortable. Know that although this is a transition you can remain on your side for a few minutes if you choose. Use your hand to press up to seated, keep your neck relaxed, teeth stay parted.

Postures savasana transitions well with:

- If you are at the end of a sequence, transition to seated to close your practice
- Closing can be as simple as taking a few deep breaths
- Hands in prayer, honouring the connection of left and right sides physically in the brain but also energetically (i.e. masculine and feminine) as well as recognizing the ability to return to the heart
- Saying a mantra or a prayer, out loud or in your head
- During practice, any reclined postures may precede or follow easily including a reclined twist, reclined moon, or supported backbends like simple supported backbend or a bridge

Physical Benefits

In savasana, the nervous system shifts deeper into a parasympathetic state, the body's rest and digest response essential for recovery. The result is a decrease in blood pressure, heart rate, muscular tension, and fatigue. The body becomes re-energized through being allowed to relax which can also improve sleep, enhance immunity, or manage chronic pain. For the brain there is an increase of theta brainwaves, associated with relaxation, creativity, and spiritual experiences.

Energetic Benefits

Practicing savasana reminds us of the importance of renewal and allowing the dead parts of ourselves to fall away. Rather than struggling to "hold on" savasana teaches us the value of letting go. This inner wisdom is connected to the 6th and 7th chakra, our energetic centers for wisdom, intuition, divine purpose, and connection to all that is.

Practicing savasana helps us understand the paradox that our place in the universe holds value yet we are also simultaneously insignificant—this posture also helps us recognize how everything is connected. It is a posture that is difficult to explain since it must be experienced wholeheartedly to truly feel its potency.

VIPARITA KARANI AKA LEGS UP THE WALL

When everything seems to be going wrong, it's legs-up-the-wall to the rescue. This posture is known for its ability to instantly ground when the world seems chaotic. As a gentle inversion this posture has many healing benefits physiologically but also energetically. It is also the only inversion recommended to those who are menstruating, given the hips are not raised by any additional props.

Proceed With Caution...

With any conditions of the spine (ex: scoliosis, lordosis, kyphosis, spondylosis)

How long?

The length of time this posture lasts fluctuates, depending exclusively on comfort. There are variations that can feel amazing for 20 minutes or more, while for others only 5 – 10 minutes is best. Typically, anywhere from 5 – 30 minutes can work well in a sequence.

Props

There are no props that are essential to this posture there is wall space it can be practiced anywhere, with or without a mat—given the floor is made of soft material like carpet.

One of my favourite variations doesn't even use a wall. It requires a bolster or pillows stacked on top of a couch, using the couch for leg support instead of the wall.

. . .

Suggested props:

Bolster

- Can stack two or three bolsters against the wall then set your sit bones on the bolster instead of directly on the wall. Ideal when hamstrings need more space or when you experience tingling/numbness in feet or toes with other variations
- For an elevated legs up the wall place bolster underneath hips (consider conditions to proceed with caution)

Blanket

- mild blanket roll underneath neck—just enough to support the curve of the cervical spine (i.e. vertebrae in neck) with excess blanket lightly folded underneath the back of head
- blanket can rest under hips or spine if sensations are too strong on the back of the pelvis or along spinal column
- can be used overtop body for warmth

Eye pillow

- over closed eyelids
- an eye pillow in both hands (palms facing up)

Sandbag

- Overtop pelvis resting overtop from hip bone to hip bone
- One on each arm

Block

- If feet are naturally dorsiflexed (i.e. sole of foot faces entirely skywards without pointing) then a block can be placed on feet. Block should lie flat effortlessly.

Strap

- Strap is useful as a loop bound around the thighs to secure legs at hip distance apart. This allows legs to fully relax since there's no ability for legs to fall outwards. If there is a buckle ensure it does not rest directly on legs.

Variations

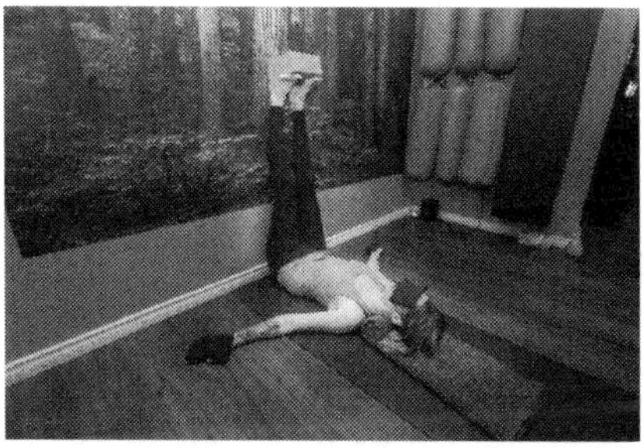

Fig. 15.2 Legs up the wall

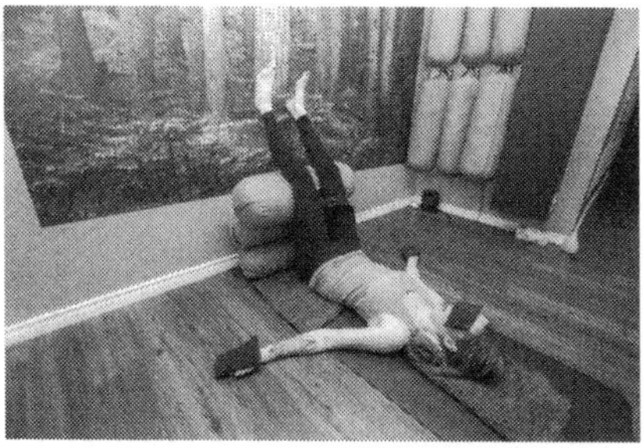

Fig. 15.3 Legs Up the Wall with Bolsters – note, pelvis is on the ground, not on a bolster (2 – 3 bolsters recommended stacked up against the wall)

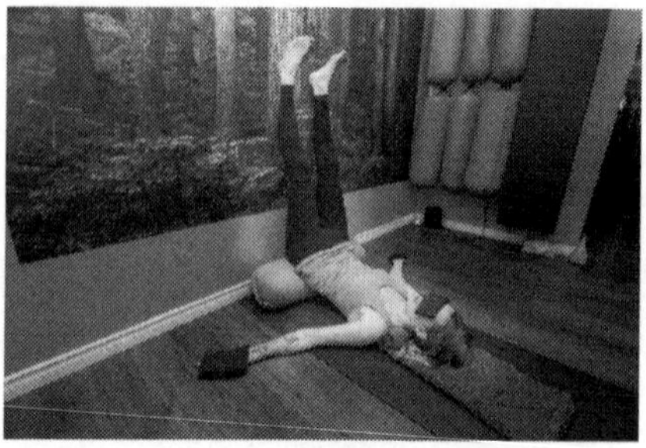

Fig. 15.4 Elevated Legs Up the Wall – hips are up on top of a bolster

Proceed with caution:

It's advised to not raise hips on a bolster under the following conditions:

- Menstruating
- Have eye (glaucoma or retinal detachment), inner ear, or sinus problems (anything that adds additional pressure to these areas)
- High Blood Pressure
- Neck or back problems—often scoliosis, kyphosis, lordosis, spondylosis, spondylolisthesis will require additional support or avoidance depending on severity

How To

Approach the wall, then slide up to the wall—or bolster— while partially lying on your side (still propped up by your elbow). Once both sit bones touch the wall, lower down beginning with your bottom shoulder then roll onto your back as legs pivot skywards.

Legs are straight but relaxed—no forcing needed—legs can rest hip distance apart or together, whatever feels more easeful.

Watch for tingling or numbness in legs which indicate nerve compression, if this occurs bend your knees and wait for the sensation to subside. The variation with bolsters stacked at the wall might be a better option to try in order to prevent any strong sensations.

Coming Out of the Posture

Bend knees, rest feet flat on the wall—option to pause during this transition, feeling the connection of your feet resting on the wall. Pay close attention to what stays grounded and what areas feel light or soft. Relax to one side with knees into chest, you are welcome to stay in this position for a few cycles of breath or as long as you need. Your head rests on an arm or directly on the mat, whatever feels best.

Postures That Transition Well

Legs-up-the-wall sequences well at the beginning or end of a class—just before savasana. Arriving at the wall can require some movement and concentration which makes it ideal to do 1st or near the end rather than in the middle of a sequence. This is also favoured energetically due to its grounding nature holding space for less clutter of the mind and assisting in our ability to "land" in the present.

Physical Benefits

Practicing this inversion assists blood in returning to the heart which can be very beneficial for the circulatory system, including blood pressure and heart health. The benefit to the circulatory system may reduce the occurrence of varicose veins and be helpful to those who stand for long periods of time—including anyone who retains water or has leg swelling. The shift in blood pressure may also assist those experiencing a headache.

For those practicing the inversion variation (with hips elevated on a bolster) there are many additional benefits to bringing the heart below the hips. Amy Matthews, a respected anatomy and movement teacher, has this to say about inversions: "We are constantly in relationship to gravity, and when we change our relationship to gravity it has an effect on our body.

Our bodies are constantly adapting to changes in our external environment and in our internal environment and seeking a dynamic and shifting state of balance, called homeostasis. A healthy circulatory system is an adaptable one—one that is able to increase and decrease blood pressure as needed. So, any activity that invites the circulatory system to adapt is one that will "improve" it, in some way.

Energetic Benefits

The grounding qualities of legs up the wall resonate with the root chakra (1st chakra) recognizing the importance of coming "home" to ourselves (more on pg 80).

When practicing variations with the hips raised it can be stimulating for the throat chakra (5th chakra) to help clarify on how to connect with our truth, radiate authenticity, and speak with confidence (more on pg 119).

Simple Supported Backbend

Some of the biggest revelations can be conveyed delicately through the practice of a gentle heart opener. A simple supported backbend can brighten up even the darkest of days. Certain life circumstances can make us feel small, while heart openers support us in feeling just how bright our light shines. When life has you feeling drained, a gentle supported backbend might be just the right reminder of the capacity that each of us has to give to the world.

Proceed With Caution...

- With any conditions of the spine (ex: scoliosis, lordosis, kyphosis, spondylosis), including just a sore, restricted, or strained lower back
- Those with eye, ear, or sinus pressure may feel better with blocks propped underneath the bolster so that your head is upright (refer to photo 15.15 for reference)

How long?

This posture can be held from 5 – 30 minutes given it is comfortable throughout the duration. Always be mindful of any tingling or numbness in arms or fingers, meaning that there's pressure on the nerves innervating the arms or hands, indicating that you must ease out of the posture.

Also be aware of any strong sensations around your spine which indicate using more support, gentler support (as in, a smaller blanket roll or bolster) or shifting out of the posture completely.

Props

An essential prop is a bolster to support underneath your back, or a rolled-up blanket, depending on which variation you choose to practice. Suggested props:

An additional bolster

- Placed underneath knees

Blanket

- Place underneath hips to reduce the curvature in the lower lumbar spine (can be useful for those with lower back conditions or pain)

Eye pillow

- over closed eyelids
- an eye pillow in both hands (palms facing up)

Sandbag

- Overtop pelvis resting overtop from hip bone to hip bone
- Resting one on each leg

Blocks can be used for variation with butterfly legs

- Underneath each knee or thigh (whatever feels more relaxing)

Strap can be used for variation with butterfly legs

- Wrapped around back, resting overtop of thighs and shins, looped underneath ankles

Variations

Simple supported backbend (using two bolsters)

How To:

Set the bolster down behind you, lengthwise. Keeping your hips grounded, bring the bolster to meet your lower back then lie down over the bolster. The back of your head rests comfortably on the bolster. Arms relaxed out to the side.

- If it feels anything less than luxurious for your lower back, set a blanket or soft block (preferably one that's low and wide) underneath your hips.
- If your head tilts too far back (rather than lying flat) place a blanket underneath the back of your head
- If it feels too far back, stack blocks underneath the bolster beneath the area around your head refer to Fig. 15.5

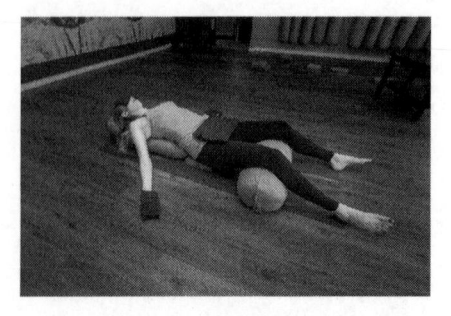

Fig. 15.5

Thoracic Fish (as a simple supported backbend) – as the name suggests this variation creates an opening through the spinal segment known as the thoracic vertebrae located in the upper back. This is often a place that closes off since many activities—including working on computers—encourage a rounding through the upper back and rolls the shoulders forward.

The energetic implications also suggest that slouching forward protects the heart from emotional turbulence—heartbreak, tough life circumstances, disappointment, and low self-worth also contribute to this stance that signals "I am closing my heart off from the world."

Practicing thoracic fish supports the healing of structural imbalances associated with this postural change as well as benefitting the heart's energetic potential to be open towards love, compassion, and forgiveness. For more information on the 4th chakra visit page 107.

- Use a gentle blanket roll so that your head rests comfortably flat on the mat or a gently folded blanket. If your head is tilted back or forward adjustment to the blanket roll is highly recommended.
- Ensure the mild blanket roll rests directly underneath the heart, resting at the largest part of the ribcage. Watch that it's not so high up the spine that it lifts the shoulders while taking care to avoid placing it beneath the lower, floating ribs.

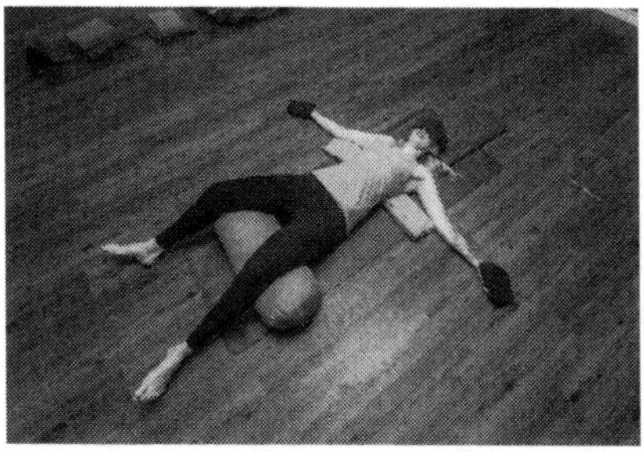

Fig. 15.6

Coming Out of the Posture

Bend knees to rest feet flat on the mat, then rest to one side—roll to lie on your side, on the floor off of the bolster (or blanket). Draw knees into chest with head flat or propped up on an arm. If the bolster is propped up on blocks: option to tuck chin into chest, lift up to rest on elbows then press up to seated.

Thoracic fish:

- Roll to one side, slide the blanket out from underneath

Postures That Transition Well

Simple supported backbends are a wonderful transition to postures on the floor. They can also be used in between a twist over a bolster or as a counterpose for a forward fold.

Physical Benefits

The opening of a simple supported backbend improves posture and can prevent or correct mild kyphosis—hunching through upper back and shoulders. A shape that decompresses the lower, lumbar spine while releasing tissue along the anterior (front) surface of the body—around the chest, shoulders, and abdomen. The openness across the front of the body, especially the abdomen as the home of the diaphragm, is useful for breathing.

Energetic Benefits

A feeling of lightening any stuck energy around the heart. This form of heart opening creates space for the radiant health of the heart chakra.

Supported Twist with a Bolster

Adding twists to your sequence has many magical properties for health and well-being. Intervertebral discs—the discs between each vertebrae—help us move, bend, and twist while absorbing the weight of gravity. Movement helps keep the discs hydrated which assists the spine in adapting to activity and preventing injury. Twists are fascinating when considering the impact of the elements—wind, earth, fire, and water—through a lens of eastern medicine.

These postures can either be heating or cooling depending on how they are practiced. In restorative yoga, applying twists to a sequence in a relaxed way supports cooling down the body by releasing excess heat as opposed to what tends to be generated through a hatha or vinyasa practice—a twist during an active posture, chair for example, would create more fire thereby increasing heat. Fire and heat can be considered physically—like during the summer months when we tend to be warmer—but also in a mental or emotional sense. If you ever find yourself steaming with anger, a twist could be the remedy to help "cool off."

This idea of keeping your cool has another layer on an energetic level. Just like wringing out a dish cloth twists are known to "wring out" any stagnant or stale energy. For this reason, it can feel very energizing afterwards, even when the posture itself is relaxing and grounding it creates space by clearing out what's no longer needed for the soul. Just as we dust out the cobwebs in our homes we can clear out the debris laying stagnant in our energetic field that must be cast out. This also makes twists a key ingredient for any change or life transition, to shed the layers that need to be released while welcoming in the positive shifts that come with new energy emerging.

Proceed With Caution...

- With any conditions of the spine (ex: disc herniation, scoliosis, lordosis, kyphosis, spondylosis)
- Neck or jaw pain

How long?

5 – 10 minutes on each side is ideal, with a counterpose in between if you feel called to do so

Props

An essential prop is a bolster to rest underneath your torso. Suggested props:

Blanket

- Place underneath the grounded hip, especially useful if you have a boney hip or are sensitive to pressure
- Placed between knees
- Rest under ankles or around feet, if you have bony ankles or are sensitive to pressure

Blocks are very useful to create more height which can relieve strain in tissues along the abdomen to increase comfort and support breathing

- One or two blocks can be used to prop up the section of bolster furthest away from you
- A soft thin block can also be useful to rest between knees

Eye pillow

- Can be placed underneath each hand

Sandbag

- Rest on top of hip that faces skywards

Variations

Although variations can be done with more/less props the shape is essentially the same.

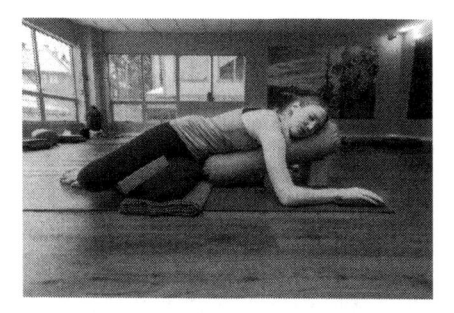

Fig. 15.7

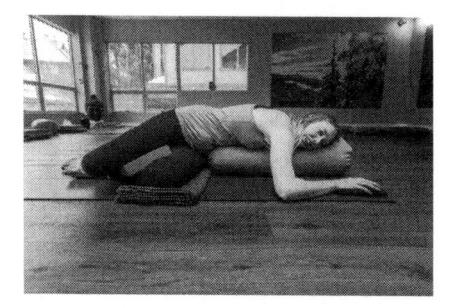

Fig. 15.8

How To

Set the bolster down, lengthwise. Bring one of your hips directly up to the bolster (one hip is grounded, the other is raised), both knees release to the side a comfortable distance apart. Place a hand on either side of your bolster, then rest your chest down. Shoulders are approximately level. Face either direction, choosing the way that it is truly comfortable for your neck.

- When one shoulder is lifted or there's any gripping in your torso (muscularly or in your breath) create more support underneath your chest i.e. prop up using blankets or use blocks underneath to make the support higher
- If this feels anything less than amazing for your neck use a blanket to prop up one side of your head to reduce the amount of rotation in neck

- For hip congestion, take knees further away from your body to increase the angle at your hip (knees will be less bent as well)

Coming Out of the Posture

Press gently down through your palms. Rise up to lift your chest away from bolster. Option to practice a counterpose:

- Knees to chest, forehead relaxed down. Shoulders relaxed, jaw is soft
- Simple supported backbend in between sides
- Regular/seated cat cow or sufi grind depending on what transitions best into the next posture (see pg 227)

Postures That Transition Well

Supported twist with a bolster transitions well with postures that also use a bolster—simple supported backbend, supported sphinx, child's pose, and forward folds.

Physical Benefits

Twists create a release for the tissues around the abdomen and spine to ensure a healthy range of motion for thoracic (upper back) and cervical (neck) vertebrae. Tension is also released in the external obliques which are involved in twisting but can also be involved in breathing.

There's a subtle opening for the intercostal muscles from the movement across the ribcage which is heavily supported by breath. Rotation of the head will create space in the tissues of the neck that help with breathing by lifting the ribcage.

Energetic Benefits

This is one of the few postures in restorative that wakes up the energy in the 3rd chakra (more on page 98). Even though the 3rd chakra is the home of fiery energy and intensity to settle into a twist in a completely relaxed and restoring way will release excess heat and fire. Releasing is a major strength of twists, especially when it comes to stagnant or stuck energy.

Just like a nice hot shower helps you feel alert and alive, twists can have a similar spiritual impact. A great option when you feel the need for energetic cleansing. This area around the abdomen is not just home to physical digestion, but spiritual digestion too! This is the place where thoughts and emotions are often processed and healthy elimination is key.

Supported Seated Angle

At first glance it's easy to miss the sweetness of supported seated angle pose. Honesty and generosity are necessary to give this posture the luxuriousness it deserves. Seeking physical depth might be tempting as strong sensations are possible to find quickly but notice how the body and mind respond when feeling out the subtle—from tissues releasing to the movement that comes with every breath. Those subtle impressions are supported by an abundance of props and mindful adjustments.

Settling into this posture means encouraging freedom throughout your hips, legs, and back which often hold stress and tension from the stress response. By taking time to unwind these areas physically, it also unravels the stress that tissues hold onto energetically. When these spaces are supported by breath it's easy to understand the charm this shape naturally holds.

Proceed With Caution...

- With any conditions of the spine (ex: disc herniation, scoliosis, lordosis, kyphosis, spondylosis)
- Groin or hamstring strain
- SI joint pain or dysfunction—taking legs closer together may make it accessible

How long?

4 – 10 minutes

Props

Two bolsters and 2 – 4 blankets. Two blocks are also recommended. This posture usually requires an abundance of props to truly relax and feel supported. Suggested props:

Blanket

- One rolled up underneath each knee, especially if there are strong sensations behind knees
- To sit on
- A blanket underneath each heel

Blocks

- Use to prop up the bolster higher. Either keep the bolster level or prop up the end furthest away from you
- A soft thin block is useful to sit on the very edge. Encourages the anterior tilt (aka forward tilt) of the pelvis which works well for forward folds, which allow for flexion at the hip

Variations

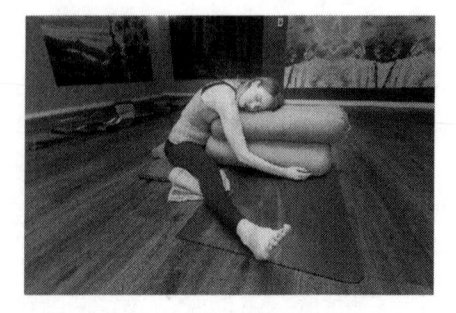

Fig. 15.9

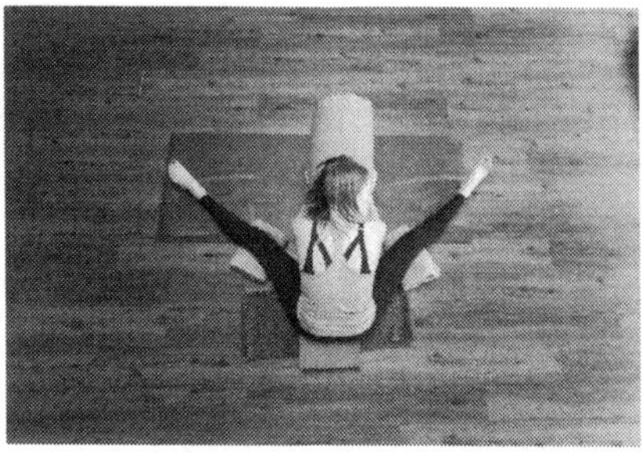

THE ENERGY & ART OF RESTORATIVE YOGA

Fig. 15.10

If forward flexion of the spine lacks the grace you deserve, a great alternative for this posture is reclined butterfly pg 50 which will allow for a similar release of the legs.

How To

Stack bolsters ahead of you, lengthwise. Apply additional props as needed.

- Blanket or block to support forward tilt of pelvis.
- Blankets under knees and feet.

Notes: if feet are not supported by blankets, ensure they are comfortable on mat

Coming Out of the Posture

- Roll up to seated. Set props aside, guide legs together
- Option to practice a counterpose
- Other options include hip movement (knees bent or legs straight) and hip circles from all fours.

Postures That Transition Well

Postures that also use a bolster. After a forward fold it can feel nice to practice a backbend or postures that allow you to lie flat.

Physical Benefits

Releases tension for adductors, hamstrings, and tissues along the back of the body.

Energetic Benefits

An opportunity to go inwards and release stored emotions that the energetic field no longer needs to hold onto. This creates space for the 2nd chakra to thrive—staying open and flexible emotionally.

Supported Crossed Leg Pose

There are unique physical and energetic benefits when practicing supported crossed leg pose. Runners and those who are active in general will particularly appreciate the physical release it creates for the gluteals, piriformis, tensor fasciae latae (TFL), and adductors. A place that tends to get "stuck" emotionally makes it a tough area to let go of tension on a physical and spiritual level. Intense thoughts and emotions regularly bubble up when practicing supported crossed legged pose. The key is to practice patience, acceptance, and love—sent intentionally into the sensations felt—to make the opening more accessible. This process of unwinding is supported by breath, notably with longer exhales or exhales out of the mouth.

Proceed With Caution...

- With any conditions of the spine (ex: disc herniation, scoliosis, lordosis, kyphosis, spondylosis)
- Groin, glute, IT band or piriformis strain.
- With any knee injuries or tweaks

How long?

4 – 8 minutes each side

Essential props:

Bolster (one, two or even three).

One or two ahead of you, or one behind you if you are lying on top

Blocks

- Set underneath knees to take pressure off of knees/ankles (can be substituted with blankets)
- Place underneath bolster for more heightA lower, wider chip block can be useful to sit on the edge of to encourage the pelvic tilt to support folding forward

Suggested props:

Blankets

- To sit on instead of a chip block
- Roll up underneath each knee as an alternative to soft blocks

For reclined variation: eye pillows

- Rest in hands, palms face skywards

Variations

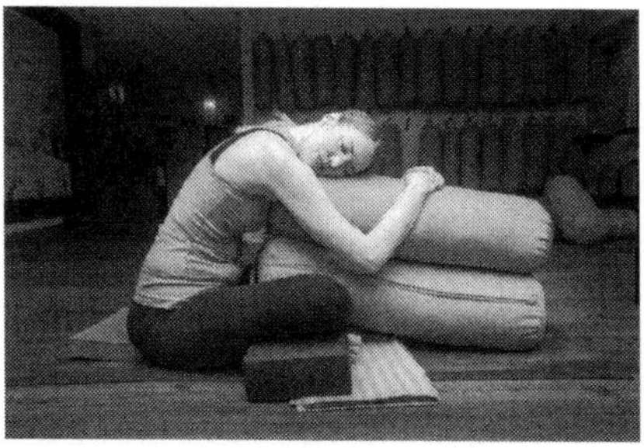

Fig. 15.11

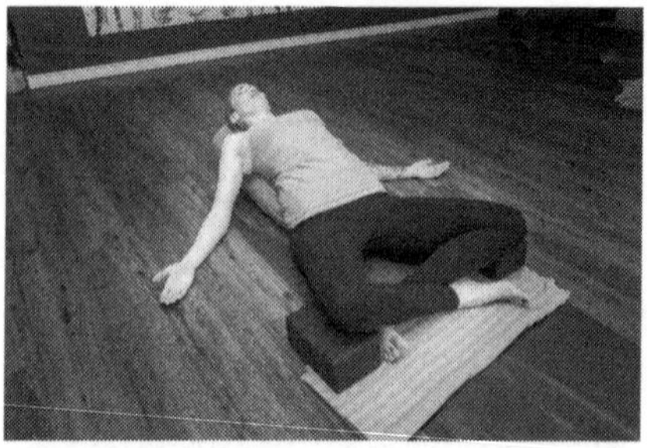

Fig. 15.12 Alternative variation lying over the bolster (generally better for those with spinal concerns)

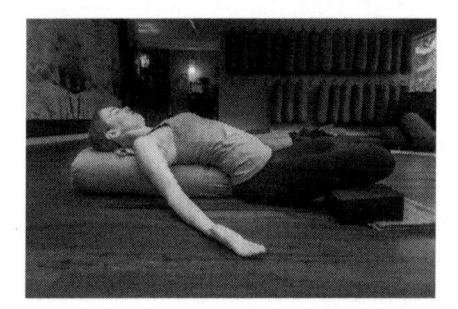

Fig. 15.13

How To

Cross one ankle in front of the other, then take your feet further away from your body. There will be space between pelvis and ankles. Shift your feet wide to rest underneath your knees (right foot will be under left knee and vise versa).

Support underneath thighs with blocks and/or blankets to take pressure off your feet and ankles. Set the bolster or bolsters ahead of you —perhaps with blocks underneath—then lay your chest on top of the props. Intensity can build quite quickly so to stay in a state of relaxation, use your props liberally!

If sensations are still very strong, lie with your bolster underneath your back like in figure 15.3 and/or take your feet closer to your body like a traditional crossed seated position in sukahsana as demonstrated in figure 2.1.

Coming Out of the Posture

- Roll up to seated, lengthen out legs. Set props aside.
- For reclined variation: uncross legs, bring them together with knees bent. Then roll to one side.

A counterpose can feel wonderful:

- Hip Movement—knees bent or legs straight
- Hip circles from all fours

Postures That Transition Well

A backbend can feel freeing afterwards: supported sphynx or a supported bridge as an example. What can be brought up mentally and emotionally during hip opening can make a twist an excellent posture to follow with energetic intent considered.

Physical Benefits

Anatomically, the illotibial tract (aka IT band) gets a bad reputation as a common site of pain, especially for runners. The location of pain isn't always the source of injury or disfunction. Contrary to popular belief the IT band does not stretch, it is thick band of connective tissue that responds to the release of the tissues attached at the origin through direct and fascial connections. By focusing on the TFL and gluteals that externally rotate the hip there will be an indirect effect on the IT band. Liberating these tissues will reduce the tension placed on the IT band which can reduce pain felt in the connective tissue or even knee pain at the attachment point.

Energetic Benefits

Energetically, the area around the pelvis is connected to the 2nd chakra. When anger, frustration, anxiety, or any other strong emotion is not fully processed this is where it gets stored. The controlling attitude of "always getting my way" will also limit openness. That mindset can be expressed in physical tightness as a response to mental or emotional inflexibility. Luckily, this is also a space that promotes freedom emotionally and energetically. When released, it invites the idea of "going with the flow" so the possibilities that life brings can be seen more clearly.

SUPPORTED CHILD'S POSE

The mythology behind child's pose speaks to the heart of the posture. A heart-warming story illustrating the importance of keeping child-like wonder while honouring divine connection. It all started with Krishna as child outside playing with his brother, Balaram. Balaram caught Krishna eating dirt so he ran to tell their mother, Yashoda. When Yashoda questioned Krishna, he denied any wrong-doing so she demanded he open his mouth to prove his innocence. When he finally complied, she didn't find any dirt only the entire universe inside of him. Even though Krishna's family knew of his divinity, his child-like form and presence made them forget. This demonstrates the importance of the willingness to be playful, curious, and interact with the world—thereby temporarily "forgetting" divinity—all the while coming back frequently to the divine nature that resides within each of us.There are circumstances in life designed to make us feel small. Child's pose, although small in stature, tells us that we can be big. This inward posture welcomes us to take a good look at the effervescence within.

Proceed With Caution...

- Knee or ankle injury, stiff ankles
- With any conditions of the spine (ex: disc herniation, scoliosis, lordosis, kyphosis, spondylosis)
- Groin or glute strain. Get extra cozy with your props!

How long?

5 – 10 minutes

Essential props:

Bolster (one or two)

- Set bolster(s) lengthwise to support underneath torso
- If there is a generous amount of space between hips and ankles, rest the bolster on heels to "sit" on the bolster

Suggested props:

Blocks

- Can be set beneath the bolster(s) to create additional height
- Shorter, wider (soft) chip block can be placed between ankles and hips if there is space between them or when hips tend to "grip"

Blankets

- Rest under knees, wedged behind the knee joint, and/or under ankles
- Use instead of the chip block to support between hips and ankles

Variations

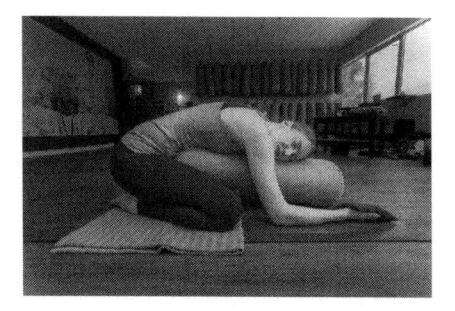

Fig. 15.14

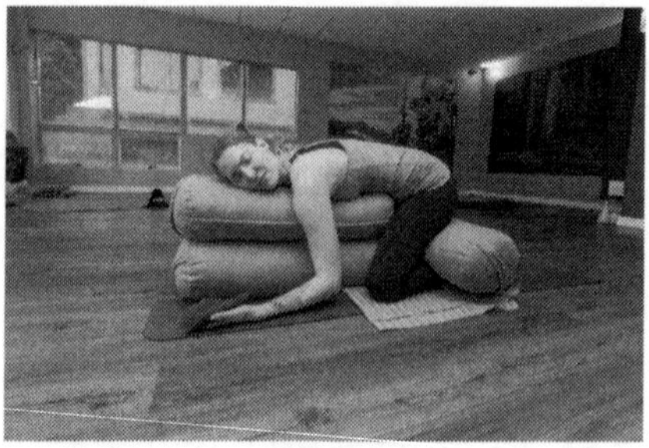

Fig. 15.15

Certain injuries don't allow for the luxurious intention of this shape, even when props are used liberally. If that is the case, the best alternative would be to practice a form of forward flexion and a hip opener. This can be one posture—supported crossed legged pose for an example—or two postures—take a forward fold followed by a reclined butterfly.

How To

Set your knees wide enough to fit a block (or bolster) between thighs. Option to use a blanket underneath knees and/or ankles. If using a block, set the bolster on top of it lengthwise. Relax your chest over the bolster. Elbows can relax out wide or tucked in and down towards your feet, whichever option feels more relaxing for your shoulders. Palms can face up or down. Be aware if there is any space between hips and ankles—use a prop to fill that space (bolster, blanket, or soft block)

Coming Out of the Posture

Roll up to seated on heels, either come up to all fours or sink hips to one side and send legs forward. A counterpose can feel wonderful.

- Knees bent, feet are wide, take both knees side to side
- Legs straight, swipe them side to side
- Hip circles from all fours or any variation cat/cow
- Sufi Grind

Postures That Transition Well

A backbend, side opening, or twist can feel amazing afterwards, especially after freeing up space around the pelvis and back. Any posture that allows for elongation of the spine can also feel soothing to practice.

Physical Benefits

Releases muscles in the groin including adductors—gracilis for example, responsible for hip adduction and assists in knee flexion. Gluteals, tissues in the back, and along the front of the ankle also receive a release.

Energetic Benefits

Benefitting the qualities of the 1st, 2nd, and even 6th chakra, child's pose gives us the chance to go inwards so we can see our potential. Just like being a fetus in the womb it can help us see where we've come from to give us an idea of where we'd like to go. The child-like wonder it brings about in a subtle way can lead to joy and buoyancy on and off the mat. For more on 1st, 2nd, and 6th chakra visit pages 84, 94, and 138 respectively.

SUPPORTED BRIDGE POSE

A beloved backbend that encourages openness for the hips and heart, supported bridge can be a heart-felt addition to any sequence.

Proceed With Caution With...

- Any inversion contraindications (heavy days of menstruation, high blood pressure or other cardiovascular health concerns, inner ear or sinus issues, glaucoma, or retinal detachment)
- Neck or shoulder injury—use blankets liberally to support
- With any conditions of the spine (ex: disc herniation, scoliosis, lordosis, kyphosis, spondylosis)

How long?

5 – 20 minutes

Essential props:

Bolsters (2 – 3 bolsters)

- One sits underneath knees, the other under pelvis

Suggested props:

Blankets

- Underneath shoulders and/or the back of your head

Eye pillows

- Over eyes
- In hands

Sandbag

- Resting across pelvis from hip bone to hip bone

Variations

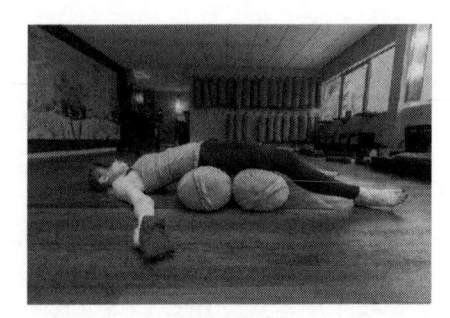

Fig. 15.16

How To

From lying down, set one bolster beneath both knees. Lift your pelvis and slide the second bolster below your hips. If your low back needs more love, stack another bolster (on top of the 1st one) underneath your legs—demonstrated in figure 15.13 for heart opening supported bridge.

Coming Out of the Posture

Set your feet back on the ground. Lift your hips, slide the bolster out from under your pelvis. Roll down to a flat back. Option for a counterpose—knees into chest or deconstructive rest pose are good options.

Postures That Transition Well

Since this posture transitions on to the floor, a reclined twist or side bend could sequence nicely. This might also be a great option right before practicing savasana.

Physical Benefits

This posture creates spinal extension, which allows for an opening through the tissues in the front of the body along the abdomen. In addition to spinal extension the cervical spine—known as the vertebrae in the neck—does the opposite by being in flexion, granting a release for the tissues along the back of the neck including the upper fibers of the trapezius and muscles involved in neck extension.

Finally, the psoas—a major hip flexor—is invited to lengthen. This large muscle tends to get tight from activity or the stress response. Since this is considered an inversion with the heart below the pelvis there may be some benefits to the adaptability of the circulatory system.

Energetic Benefits

Although this opening encourages space in the 2nd and 4th chakras related to the pelvis and heart, the warmth of this posture may also be felt energetically in the 5th (throat) or even 6th (third eye) chakras. Practicing versions—even subtle ones—encourage us to "flip our perspective" taking a deeper look at what surfaces when we settle into a meditative state. Although attaching or clinging to thoughts isn't useful neither is pushing them down. They might be coming up for a reason. This is a chance to give ourselves permission to feel without judgement while holding the space for when we're ready to let go.

Supported Heart Opening Bridge

Although the opening and intention of this posture is like a regular supported bridge there are a few glaring differences: particularly, the expansiveness through the heart. At first glance the shape might look like an intense opening but the experience can be soft and illuminating—like the warmth of coming home to a warm fire on a cold day. Some students also get nervous since it requires tedious set up with a cautious entry but once you're "there" it might become one of the postures you never want to leave.

Proceed With Caution With...

- Any conditions of the spine (ex: scoliosis, lordosis, kyphosis, spondylosis)
- Neck injury
- Eye, ear, or sinus pressure/issues

How long?

8 – 20 minutes

Essential props:

Bolster (at least 2, maybe 3)

- Rest under back and legs

Blankets (1 – 3)

- Folded to support head, neck, and shoulders

Strap

- To bind legs so they stay on the bolster

Suggested props:

Extra blankets

- Under head/neck/shoulders

Eye pillows

- Over eyes
- In hands whether they are facing up or down

Sandbag

- Set across the front of pelvis (from hip to hip)

Variations

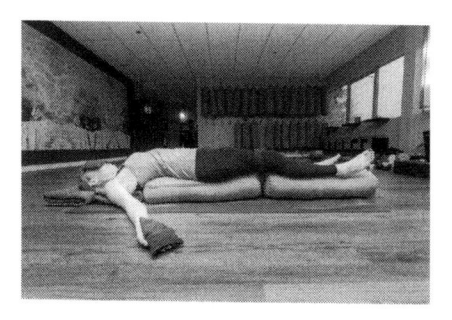

Fig. 15.17

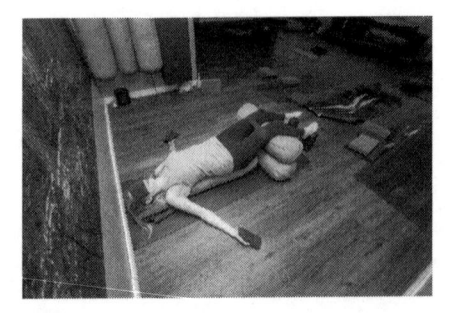

Fig. 15.18 The perfect variation if your lower back needs extra TLC. In this variation, instead of the far bolster resting straight ahead of you, turn and stack.

How To

Set one bolster down, lengthwise on your mat and sit down on top of it. Secure your strap around your legs somewhere between knees and hips—the buckle is between your thighs rather than against your body. Place folded blankets on the mat behind the bolster. Set the next bolster (or 2 stacked bolsters) so bolsters line up end-to-end.

Lie down on top of the bolster so your shoulders roll off the end. Legs rest either over a single bolster lengthwise or on top of two stacked bolsters that lie across your mat. Make sure head is level—if you find it's tilting back it's a great place to add more blankets, if your head tilts forward adjust the blankets so they are level.

Coming Out of the Posture

Slide your feet off to one side (all the way off of the bolster) then roll the rest of your body to the same side. Draw knees into chest, round your spine. Staying for 5 – 10 breaths on your side is optional and can make an excellent counterpose. Then remove any straps before moving on. Other counterposes include resting on back with knees into chest, constructive rest pose, or savasana.

Postures That Transition Well

Since you are already lying down after coming out of the posture this might be the perfect shape to practice before savasana. Alternatively, it can transition well into any reclined position or seated postures. After freeing up space across the chest and abdomen a forward fold, twist, or hip opener can sequence well.

Physical Benefits

The expansiveness created across the chest makes this perfect posture to open through the pectoral muscles. In addition, this is one of the few postures that has significant extension through the upper thoracic vertebrae which also support the intervertebral joints of that area. The neck flexion experienced releases tissues in the upper back—the upper fibers of the trapezius—and other tissues located in the back of the neck typically associated with neck extension.

Although it is still considered an inversion—that still have specific effects including increasing pressure in the head meaning to proceed with caution with head injury, eye/ear/sinus problems—it's one of the few inversions that can feel good to practice during menstruation. If your digestion is slightly "off" it is one of the few inversions to foster a positive experience.

Energetic Benefits

With very similar energetic benefits to supported bridge (more on pg 180) this variation is like sending energetic jumper cables straight to the heart—without an abrupt shock. If your heart needs a spiritual boost to support you in forgiveness, love—to yourself or others—or tapping into your compassionate qualities, this posture is where it's at. It'll break you open in the most compassionate and loving way.

With neck flexion there is also a deeper connection to the qualities of the throat chakra (more on pg 118) which speak to the feelings of freedom nurtured in this shape. Being able to speak our truth, lovingly yet unapologetically, is our birth right. Honing in on the potential to recognize and honour our truth is the first step towards living by it whole-heartedly.

. . .

Supported Bound Angle Pose

This posture is a wonderful option that includes an opening for the inner thighs, a place often in need of a bit of extra love anatomically and spiritually. Active go-getters will appreciate the subtle release in the adductors while on an energetic level this shape encourages shifts for the 2nd chakra related to emotional stability and fluidity.

One of the best parts about this posture is the level of openness it encourages for the energetic spaces that tend to close off during heavy life circumstances. When practicing with a bolster under the spine this posture also acts as a gentle heart opener. This chakra pairing is a powerhouse couple to experience emotional freedom and stability. The hips and the heart are places we deserve to feel open and safe—this posture aligns directly with that intention. It also shows us that opening these areas doesn't have to be forceful to be powerful. Supported bound angle reminds us that being "cracked open" can have a warmth that feels subtle, tender, and loving.

Proceed With Caution...

- Sacroiliac joint pain— it may help you to place your feet further away
- Any conditions of the spine (ex: disc herniation, scoliosis, lordosis, kyphosis, spondylosis)
- Adductor strain

How long?

5 – 25 minutes

Essential props:

Either a bolster or two blocks

- If using a bolster; it is set underneath both knees, or one under each thigh or knee
- When using blocks, rest them underneath knees or thighs

Suggested props:

Bolster

- Underneath your back to pair it with a simple supported backbend variation
- Use beneath knees instead of using blocks

Blankets

- Underneath your back and/or hips
- Can be used as substitutes for blocks under knees/thighs
- Place underneath ankles for added comfort
- If lying flat, it's recommended to use half a blanket roll to support underneath your neck and use the other half lightly folded under the back of your head

Eye pillow

- Relaxed over eyes
- Resting in hands, palms flipped open
- Strap (only for simple supported backbend variation with bolster beneath back—not appropriate when lying flat)
- Wrapped around lower back, overtop thighs and shins, then wrapped underneath ankles

Ensure the buckle does not rest on the body and that the strap is taught so that it provides subtle support for the legs and decompresses the lower back.

Variations

The variation depends on the props used—all of them involve using butterfly legs in a diamond shape. The depth and sensation will change with the amount of props used and how they are applied. In both variations demonstrated below, a bolster is used. In the first and

2nd photo, the bolster is propped up by additional blocks. However, supported bound angle can be practiced with just one bolster (demonstrated in the 3rd photo) or no bolster at all.

Exploring a range of shapes and staying curious is encouraged as each variation will create a slightly different experience on a physical and energetic level. Note: variation using a strap does require support underneath your back (a bolster is ideal).

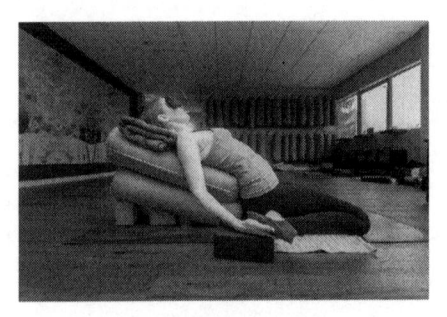

Fig. 15.19

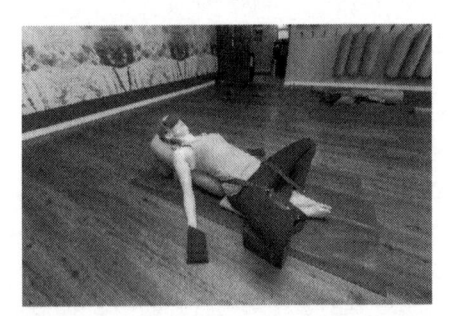

Fig. 15.20 Supported Bound Angle with additional blocks underneath for more height (figure above and below.)

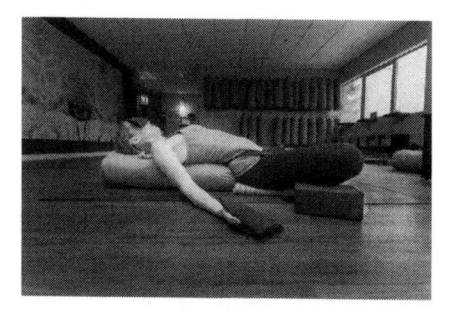

Fig. 15.21 Supported Bound Angle with no blocks underneath the bolster (additional extension for the lower lumbar spine)

How To

Make sure blocks are close by (before lowering down). (You might even set them up first, then readjust when lying down) If you are using a bolster, set it down behind you so that it touches your lower back. Lie down on your back (or bolster, readjusting as needed). Set blocks (or a bolster, wide across the mat) underneath both knees or thighs for support.

Coming Out of the Posture

Transitions out of any posture can be easeful when we are fully present with how our body responds to certain actions. For instance, if you are using blocks stacked under a bolster that supports your back it might be easier to tuck your chin to chest and rise up to seated. This wouldn't be the same circumstance for a bolster that lies flat or if you're flat on your back. In that case, gathering your thighs with your hands and drawing them together to roll off to one side would be easeful. We might be used to making life hard, but this is the chance for simplicity! Make it the most comfortable, relaxed transition you can. Facilitate that ease by staying connected to your breath. Take your time, and enjoy each moment even if it takes 5 – 10 breaths to arrive there. Sometimes, the longer it takes the sweeter it feels.

Counterpose options:

- Before rolling to one side, take deconstructive rest pose

- Hip movement with knees bent

Postures That Transition Well

Depending on the variation, if you're transitioning to the floor a reclined twist, reclined moon, supported side opening, or simple supported thoracic fish would transition well. From seated, a posture that uses a forward fold sequences nicely.

Physical Benefits

Release for the adductor group in your legs. With simple supported backbend it allows for an opening through your chest and shoulders (pectorals) and creates space along the anterior surface of the body.

Energetic Benefits

Check out page 88 for more information on the 2nd chakra. With simple supported backbend can also connect to the 4th chakra, more on page 108.

Side Lying Release

Releasing the tissue around the ribcage is essential for breathing. When ribcage movement is limited due to tightness, so is respiration. Freedom to breathe easefully supports the relaxation response in the nervous system. On an energetic level, the ribs protect vital organs, specifically the area around the heart. Dr. Joe Dispenza asserts that the heart produces a magnetic field up to 3 meters wide. In fact, the heart produces the largest rhythmic electromagnetic field of any of the body's organs, making it the most powerful generator of electromagnetic energy in the body. Creating movement and freedom in this area, for body and breath, has a direct effect on our energetic field. When breath flows easily, so does prana—the life force energy that drives us.

Proceed With Caution With...

- Healing rib fracture

- Shoulder injury
- Neck injury - support your head during the posture and for transitions into and out of

How long?

4 – 10 minutes each side

Essential props:

Blanket

- Rolled or folded resting under the largest part of your ribs (fold or roll based on preference)

Suggested props:

Additional blankets

- Resting under the side of your head
- Placed between your thighs or knees
- If lying on your side is less than cozy, lay a soft blanket down to rest under the length of your body

Eye pillows

- Resting in hands and/or between elbows

Sandbag

- Relaxed over the side of your hip that faces skywards

Soft, chip block

- Can be used instead of a blanket to support head or rest between thighs/knees.

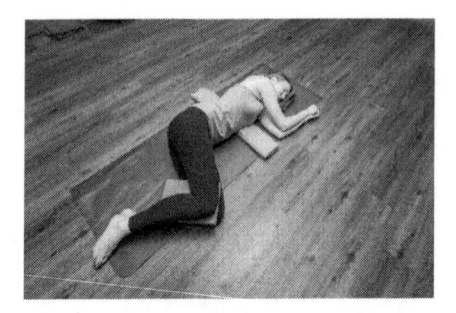

Fig. 15.22

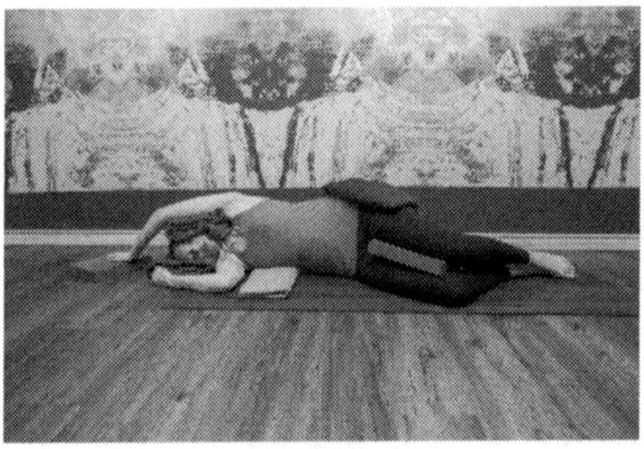

Fig. 15.23

Variations

Turn to one side, with knees bent (slightly or deeply, whatever your preference). Set your rolled or folded blanket underneath the largest part of your ribs. Watch that it's not so low that it presses on your lower, floating ribs but also not so high that it rests at your shoulder. Head can rest on your arm or a blanket/soft block. If any strong sensations arise, adjust your blanket roll/fold.

Coming Out of the Posture

Slide the blanket roll out from under your ribs, take time to rest on your side and notice how the side of your body feels.

Postures That Transition Well

Since this posture brings you directly onto your side it makes it easy to transition to many shapes, either seated or lying down. Since the blanket is already under your ribcage it can transition well to thoracic fish effortlessly.

Physical Benefits

The intercostals muscles are known as the muscles between each rib that create lift during a normal inhalation and draw the ribs down during a strong exhalation. When these muscles are released, breathing becomes enhanced. Shallow, quick breathing can prompt the sympathetic nervous system (stress response) while slow, deep breathing allows for the parasympathetic (relaxation) response to work its' magic.

Energetic Benefits

Supporting health breathing isn't just for physical health—our energetic field thrives from an enhanced flow of prana. The heart chakra also benefits from opening the spaces around the ribs.

Reclined Side Lying Release

Grounded, expansive, and sustainable—this posture is everything you'd hope for in a side opening.

Proceed With Caution With...

- With any conditions of the spine (ex: scoliosis, lordosis, kyphosis, spondylosis)
- Any issue with ribs—might be helpful to keep arms down

How long?

4 – 10 minutes each side

Props:

This shape often doesn't require props however, when practicing the variation with arms overhead blankets can be very supportive. Most students cannot take their arms overhead without hovering their arms. Using blankets takes the muscular effort out of the arms.

Suggested props:

Blankets

- Resting beneath arms and/or shoulders if arms are overhead

Sandbag

- Set across the front of pelvis between hip bones

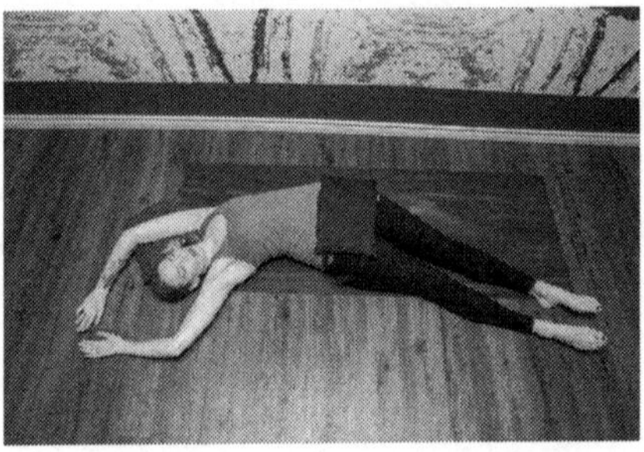

Fig. 15.24

Variations

From lying down, keep legs straight and walk the heels a few inches over to one side. Curve your upper body over in the same direction (creating a moon shape) while both hips stay anchored. If you choose to take arms overhead be mindful of any strong sensations in your shoulders, if they need extra love use blankets to support under arms (if arms hover, place support underneath). Otherwise, arms rest at your sides or palms on belly—especially if it feels anything less than amazing for your shoulders. Most athletes, particularly those with strong shoulders, will appreciate using blankets for extra lift under the arms or practicing an alternative arm placement.

Coming Out of the Posture

Walk everything back to center (savasana). Can feel soothing to do a counterpose between sides and/or afterwards. Knees into chest or savasana are good choices.

Postures That Transition Well

Transitioning into other postures on the floor can be convenient—a twist, a supported bridge, or supported bound angle for example. Might also be a great posture to practice before savasana.

Physical Benefits

An opening through the side of the body is one of the notable benefits of this shape. This creates space in the intercostal muscles which are known as accessory muscles for breathing. This opening along the side also creates sensation for tissues around your hip (on the opened side) including the psoas. Releasing this hip flexor may result in relief for other areas of the body.

A tight psoas can create serious postural problems—causing anterior (forward) pelvic tilt—that can result in lower back pain. Those who suffer from back pain may see improvement by practicing this form of opening. There is also a subtle opening for the tensor fascae latae (TFL), a muscle that feeds into the iliotibial (IT) band—a thick band of connective tissue that attaches to the lateral condyle of the tibia on the outside of the knee.

Therefore, a tight TFL can result in increased tension for the IT band which can contribute to knee pain or dysfunction. Releasing the TFL prevents and supports healing for knee pain related to the IT band while contributing to healthy knee function. Lastly, the lateral flexion in this posture also allows the obliques, quadratus lumborum, and erector spinae to lengthen along the open side.

Energetic Benefits

A beautiful characteristic of this posture is the overwhelming support the earth provides—making it a magnet for nurturing qualities of the root chakra. In addition to its grounding qualities, the energy of the hips and heart also play a role. In fact, when practiced in such a grounded way the 2nd and 4th chakra characteristics can smoothly assist one another. Coming from a place of stability is exceptionally valuable when dealing with emotional matters that step forward in these energetic spaces.

The 4th chakra holds the space to give and receive love, a gift that only develops with the help of 2nd chakra by forming relationships. Not surprisingly, the sacral chakra is involved with how we experience pleasure while the heart leans in to how we embrace joy. By approaching these complementary gifts with a strong, stable foundation building upon them becomes seamless.

Reclined Hero Pose

Hero pose has an inspiring origin story. The mythology involves Hanuman, a fierce warrior of the monkey army. He befriended King Ram who was married to Sita. One day, an evil demon grew jealous of Ram and Sita's love, prompting him to steal Sita away to his island kingdom. Ram sent his trusted friend Hanuman to save her. He arrived at the coast near where Sita had been captured. He knelt down and prayed he would be given the grace to do the impossible.

When he felt as though he had called in enough energy, he pressed his feet into the ground with such force that it sent a shockwave through the land—knocking down trees and hills around him. He took this strength to leap over the ocean to rescue Sita. His unwavering strength, faith, and bravery serves as an inspiration to follow in our practice.

The true bravery in a restorative hero pose is in connecting to our truth. Courage is derived from caring less about the "look" of the posture and more about the experience. We must also have faith in our decisions regarding the variation we take—that same faith can be guidance to come out of the posture if it doesn't align with our intention of relaxation. By seeing postures as a stepping stone to a deeper experience we can appreciate the subtle sensations. Rather than suffer in pain we all deserve to experience bliss.

Proceed With Caution With...

- Knee injury
- Ankle injury
- Low back issues with the reclined variation

How long?

4 – 10 minutes each side

Props:

Remember, the aim is for subtle sensation rather than intensity. Ultra-bendy students not use as many props but for the majority of the population, the more the merrier! Even students who identify as flexible or open can benefit from using more props than they expect.

Essential props:

One of two bolsters (depending on whether reclining or not)

- Supports your back, either sitting up or reclining

Blankets

- Underneath knees and/or ankles

Block (large or chip)

- To sit on (rests under sit bones)

Suggested props:

- Additional blankets

Resting under lower back or head

- Eye pillows

Over eyes

- Sandbag

Resting over your legs

Variations

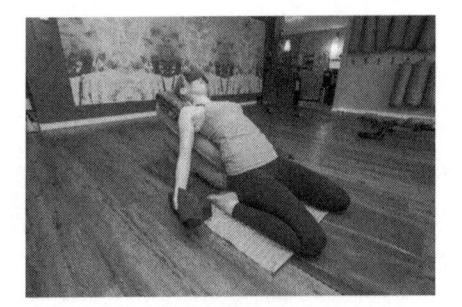

Fig. 15.25

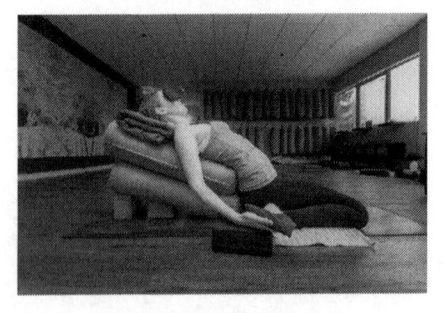

Fig. 15.26 Reclined Hero Pose

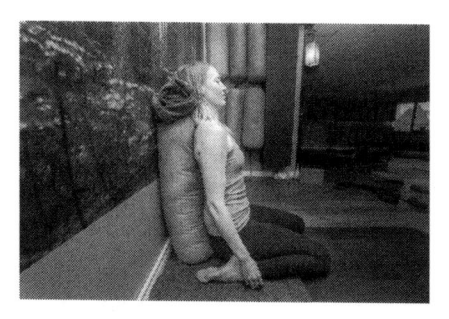

Fig. 15.27 Supported Hero Pose (at the wall)

How To

Start by kneeling on padding that rests under knees and/or the tops of your feet. With hips raised (from kneeling)—knees set hip distance apart or together—use your hands to widen the space just below your knees (i.e. the backs of your calves in your lower leg) Sit down on your block or blanket. For variation at wall, rest bolster behind your back against the wall. A blanket fold or roll may be needed for taller individuals to support behind the head.

For reclined variation, have blocks, blankets, and bolsters ready. Prop up using bolsters (and blocks potentially) then lie down on top. If your head tilts back a lot, prop up your head with a blanket. Go luxuriously slow into this posture to figure out what depth will allow for true relaxation. Have an abundance of props ready and use them liberally.

Coming Out of the Posture

For reclined posture: tuck chin into chest first, then lift up to seated. All variations, rise up to all fours.

A counterpose is a welcomed option:

- Cat/cow or variations
- Pedal out legs from all fours

Postures That Transition Well

A forward fold can sequence nicely after the length and space for the lower back. After a generous amount of counterposing for knees and ankles child's pose can feel amazing, especially after a reclined variation to lengthen out your back. Anything that transitions gracefully to all fours—supported twist with a bolster or sphynx for example—can sequence well.

Physical Benefits

Quadricep femoris as the "quad" suggests is a group of 4 muscles. Vastus lateralis, vastus medialis, vastus intermedius, and the rectus femoris originate on the femur (leg) bone and attach on the patella (knee cap). Restorative variations of heros pose allow for an opening for this muscle group in a gentle, supportive way.

Reclined options will also create length for the psoas, a deep hip flexor. The intensity of the stress response often gets stored here since it's a muscle responsible for acting on "fight" or "flight."

Energetic Benefits

Our legs carry us through life—the good, the bad, and the ugly. Releasing the quadricep group it can bring up a lot of emotional energy—helping us realize we don't have to carry all of life's burdens. Letting go of the stored energy in these tissues is a way of "walking off" anything holding us back so we can stride proudly into the future.

The psoas release has a powerful energetic intention. It's known as the "muscle of the soul" the energy of the stress response often gets stored here. Reclined variations are naturally like soul food when paired with conscious breathing. The psoas responds well physically and energetically to a gentler, nourishing approach. Intensity and force will only create more tension in the long run. By easing into this shape and supporting the opening with breath, the psoas is given an opportunity to release any stored energetic intensity buried in the tissue.

. . .

Reclined Twist

With a heart opened skywards and an openness across the chest there are clear reasons why a reclined twist feels so sweet. This variation is also the most grounded twist, meaning it has the most connection to the earth itself. When thoughts are buzzing around wildly this grounding posture can give you the gift of landing right back into the present.

Proceed With Caution With...

- With any conditions of the spine (ex: scoliosis, lordosis, kyphosis, spondylosis)
- Shoulder injury—make sure your shoulder is supported. Perhaps more support under knees is also helpful

How long?

4 – 10 minutes each side

Props:

A reclined twist does not necessarily "need" any props—especially if you are the ultra bendy type—however the goal is to be completely comfortable. Release any shame you feel about supporting yourself and be open to make this an indulgent shape to practice. Be aware if any body parts tend to hover or if your breath feels restricted in any way, those are signals to be more generous with props.

Suggested props:

Blankets

- Resting under the grounded hip and leg
- Between your knees or thighs
- Underneath both thighs

Eye pillows

- In hands opened skywards

Sandbag

- Resting on top of your hip

Strap

- Bind legs (remove strap before transitioning to the other side)

Variations

The variations for this posture are not about changing the shape itself, rather it involves moving the body to increase, decreases or change the sensation.

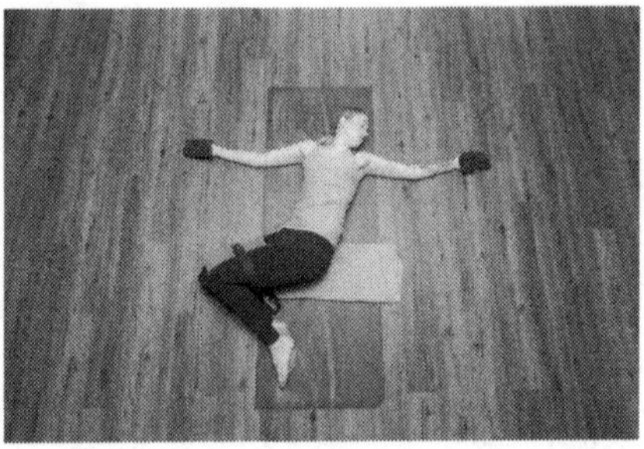

Fig. 15.28

How To

From lying down, draw knees towards chest, relax arms out wide, palms face up or down. Relax your knees to one side, send your gaze in the opposite direction. Foot or knee placement will affect how this shape is experienced. Generally, knees further away from the body will decrease sensation whereas taking feet further away may feel more stable but will likely increase sensation across the top hip. These choices of knee and foot placement are based on preference. Feel free to experiment with what is comfortable.

To hip shift, or not to hip shift?

This debate is an interesting one with some strong arguments from yoga teachers and dedicated practitioners on either side. What is meant by "hip shift" is the option to pick up your hips and shift them to the opposite side before your knees lower down. As an example, if your knees were going to the right, you would pick up your hips to shift them to the left before knees relax to the side.

Rather than label either option as "right" or "wrong" consider this an invitation to try both. Each option will have slightly different sensations to offer. Luckily, both can be practiced safely with a healthy dose of curiosity.

Coming Out of the Posture

Release any props around legs (i.e. blanket from between thighs or strap around legs). Guide one leg back to center, followed by the other. Great place to hug knees into chest to either a.) stay still b.) create movement. Gentle circles with knees, rocking side to side, whatever gentle movement calls to you

Postures That Transition Well

Since the twist is already on the ground, using this as your last posture before savasana might be a great option—especially considering the grounding nature of this pose. Other floor-based postures also transition well. The other nice aspect of this pose is that you can always roll all the way to one side as your transition to rise up to seated—making it effortless. So to practice seated postures is also accessible with no fuss.

Energetic Benefits

Shares many of the benefits with supported twist with a bolster but with a few key differences energetically. Supported twist with a bolster feels more closed off energetically which is very valuable when turning inwards, whereas reclined twist is much more open on an energetic level.

There is no "better" option energetically, just one that aligns more out of what you need to lean into. One is liberating the other introspective. One is more buoyant, the other grounding. Determine your energetic needs for the day then choose your ideal twist accordingly.

Reclined twist is a bit of a paradox energetically since it is so grounded and stable—associated with the 1st chakra—but also so open and bright to resonate with the upper chakras. Perhaps it is a sign that we could all use a little more of this balance in our lives.

SUPPORTED SPHYNX

Something to love about supported sphynx is the ability to cultivate openness while being given permission to go inwards. This shape has a very introspective quality yet encourages an opening around the heart—showing us we can be open and receptive while giving ourselves space.

Proceed With Caution With...

- With any conditions of the spine (ex: scoliosis, lordosis, kyphosis, spondylosis)
- Breast tenderness—a good alternative would be a supported bridge or supported heart-opening bridge

How long?

5 – 12 minutes

Essential props:

Bolster or Rolled Blanket

- Supported under chest

Block or rolled blanket

- For forehead to rest on

Suggested props:

Blankets

- Under hip bones

To place on top of the block under forehead (to make it softer)

Eye pillows

- In hands whether they are facing up or down

Sandbag

- Placed across lower back or the backs of legs

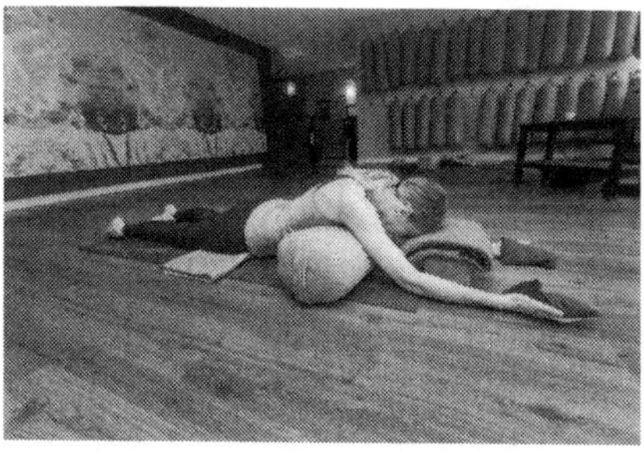

Fig. 15.29

Variations

Set your bolster or rolled blanket down across the mat. Lower your elbows ahead of the bolster, then bring hips all the way down. Set support underneath forehead. Elbows can rest wide or further away (without propping up the body—let the bolster do the work!)

Coming Out of the Posture

Raise your head up, slide the bolster out from under your chest. Lower all the way down onto your belly. Lying flat for 5 – 10 cycles of breath can feel incredible after this posture. Absorb and experience the shifts in your body, breath, and energetic presence.

Postures That Transition Well

After coming out of sphynx it's very easy to transition to other prone (lying on belly) postures or to roll over into supine (facing up on your back) making many other postures easy to access. From prone, rolling to one side then transitioning up to seated can also be easeful.

Physical Benefits

The shape of sphynx encourages healthy mobility for the intervertebral joints between each vertebra. This supports maintaining healthy range of motion with the extension of the lumbar spine and some of the lower thoracic vertebrae. There is an opening for the tissues of the abdomen and chest. Space is also created for the psoas, a deep hip flexor that is often contracted during the "fight or flight" response—a very important area to receive attention.

Energetic Benefits

Backbends help us transcend the habitual patterns that obscure the light of our soul. There are certain situations in life that cause us to recoil and protect ourselves from pain and suffering. Although that can be useful for a limited amount of time, long term fosters feelings of isolation and despair. Backbends gift us the freedom to stay open even after painful events.

A unique benefit of sphynx is the effect of gravity around the abdomen. As a society we are so used to being told to "suck in" or feel ashamed of our belly. In this posture, let your breath flow easily and let go of any tension or shame associated with that space. For muscles to work effectively they need relaxation between contractions so rather than an ab work out, consider this a "work in"—physically and mentally.

SUPPORTED SEATED FORWARD FOLD

In this introspective posture learn to "tune out the world" while receiving insight into your inner workings. Certain postures are confronting mentally and emotionally—supported forward fold tends to fall into that camp. Energetically, a forward fold makes us take a good hard look at ourselves. This is where certain fears—judgment, skepticism, unworthiness—stare you down. While on some level that might seem terrifying, we are asked to lean into what creates freedom.

Rather than get frustrated or angry, perhaps it is a better question to consider: why are these bubbling up? And, is it time to let these go? Perhaps these weren't stored in our tissues or in the back of our mind to taunt us, rather they are there to help us grow and become more present. When we break down the barriers of who we "aren't" the space is created to understand and feel beneath the surface, uncovering who we truly are.

Proceed With Caution With...

- Any conditions of the spine (ex: scoliosis, lordosis, kyphosis, spondylosis)
- Hamstring injury
- Lower back issues/injury

How long?

5 – 10 minutes

Essential props:

Two bolsters (or one bolster and a rolled blanket)

- rests underneath your knees (or a rolled blanket)

- supports beneath your chest

Two blocks

- To prop up the bolster under your chest

Suggested props:

Blankets (or chip block)

- To rest under head
- For sitting on to encourage the anterior (forward) pelvic tilt

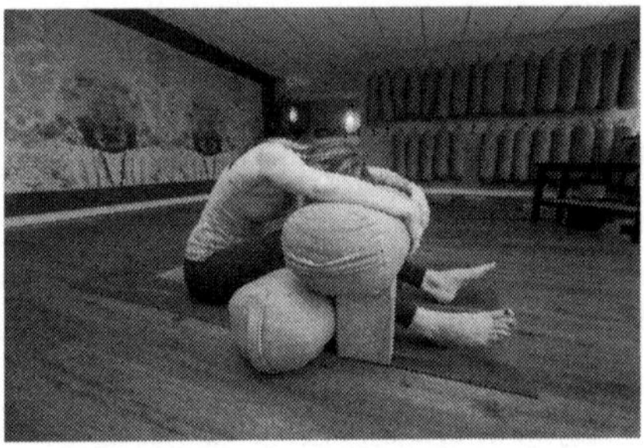

Fig. 15.30

Variations

The variation below demonstrates the posture with three bolsters. A great choice for the lower back and legs when they need freedom from struggle. This variation provides more space to open up in a relaxed way.

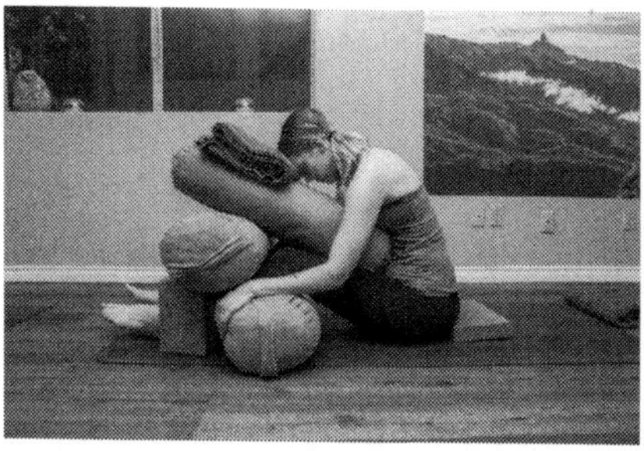

Fig. 15.31

How To

Set bolster (or rolled blanket) underneath both knees, place one block on the outside of each shin. Stack 2nd bolster on top of blocks then drape yourself over the bolster. Make sure your head is supported (rather than hanging out in space) which might mean using a blanket or a 3rd bolster.

Coming Out of the Posture

Roll up (head is heavy so it comes up last)

Postures That Transition Well

Backbends can feel wonderful after practicing a forward fold. Other great options are postures that lengthen your spine—side lying release for example.

Physical Benefits

This posture is lengthening for the hamstring group along the backs of the upper legs. This group is made up of three muscles: semitendinosis, semimembranosis, and bicep femoris. Forward folds also releases tissues along the back like the erector spinae.

Energetic Benefits

The hamstrings are another major muscle group that hold tension from preparing the body to "fight or flee" due to the stress response.

Creating space for these muscles can unwind the stored energy in these tissues. Intense emotions—fear, anger, frustration, despair—are given a healthy outlet to be set free. Energetically, the back of the body leans towards issues from our history. Letting go of the stored energy in these tissues is a way of "walking off" the energetic residue of the past that doesn't resonate with your present self.

Louise Hay shares valuable information about energetic blockages in the back. She asserts the lower back relates to fears around money while middle back relates to guilt and upper back speaks to a lack of emotional support. If these sensations bubble up physically or mentally consider how affirmations can support your practice. Repeating words like "I am supported," "Life supports and loves me," or "I am abundant." Focusing with breath allows prana—the life force with the potential to heal—is sent directly into these spaces.

ADVASANA AKA REVERSE SAVASANA

Advasana is a great alternative to practicing a conventional savasana when lying down on your back is not accessible. It's also a wonderful pose to practice on its own. There's a level of ease to lean into that makes this shape feel like comfort food for the soul. For many people it's a sleeping position so settling in on the mat seems like second nature.

Proceed With Caution With...

- Neck issues
- Groin strain
- Pregnancy—propping up the bent leg and lying on a blanket may make this more approachable
- Breast tenderness

How long?

4 – 8 minutes each side

Props

This shape often doesn't necessarily require props if you have a very generous cushion on your mat. Blankets add a bit of extra luxury so they come highly recommended.

Suggested props:

Blankets

- Placed under hips and the leg with knee bent
- Rolled up and place under inner thigh of bent knee
- Underneath side of head

Soft chip block

- Can be used instead of a blanket underneath inner thigh and/or under bent knee

Eye pillow

- In outstretch arm or threaded variation

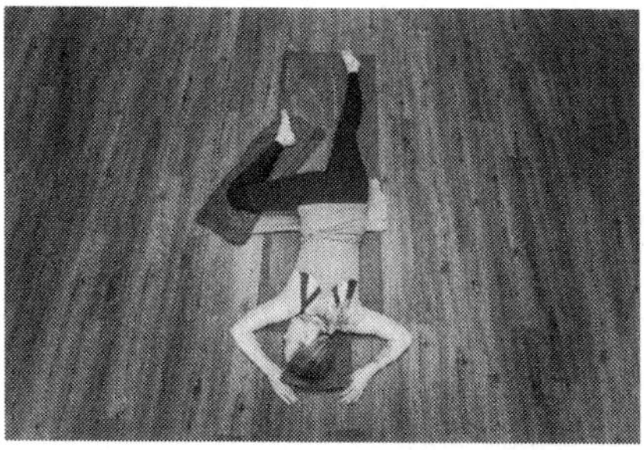

Fig. 15.32

Variations

The threaded variation below demonstrates a perfect option if your chest feels less than comfortable in the original pose. To practice, thread your outside arm all the way across to the opposite side of your mat. Be conscious of any shoulder sensitivity. Use a generous blanket fold under your head.

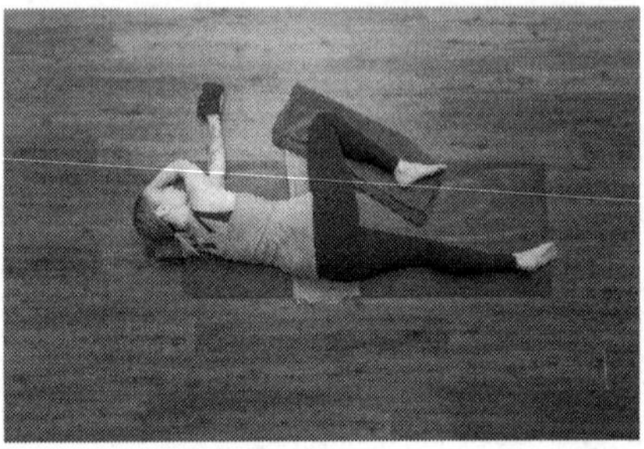

Fig. 15.33

How To

Have one blanket underneath both hips in prone (lying on your belly) then slide one knee towards the upper corner of your mat. Option to place another blanket or prop under raised knee. Turn your head to face the same direction. Arms can rest wherever they are the most comfortable. Suggestions: around your head with elbows bent or thread your bottom arm across (especially if there is chest tenderness).

Coming Out of the Posture

Slide your leg with the bent knee back down your mat. For potential counterpose: stay still while lying prone or rock hips side to side. If transitioning onto back, keep knee bent, roll over then hug knees into chest or take feet wide and alternate with knees side to side.

Postures That Transition Well

This posture can transition easefully either onto the back for reclined postures or rolling up onto your side to rise up to all fours. Could sequence into child's pose, sphynx or supported twist with a bolster.

. . .

Physical Benefits

An opening for the inner thigh—the adductor group. Depending on where arms are placed can also create space across the chest (pectorals). Head rotation releases muscles in the neck involved in rotation like the sternocleidomastoid and scalenes.

Energetic Benefits

Advasana emanates qualities of the 1st chakra due to the significant connection with the earth yet it also leans into the resources of the 2nd chakra. Louise Hay has interesting thoughts to share on the energetic repercussions of the hips. She maintains that the hips carry the body in perfect balance, granting major thrusts to propel us forward in the right direction. Hip dysfunction or chronic tension may relate to a fear of moving forward, thinking there's nothing to move forward to.

Questions to ask yourself would look like: "what would I do if fear wasn't an option?" or "am I living my life to its fullest potential?" and even "am I seeing the life the way it really is?" Understanding that life always has opportunities to look forward to is part of healing this misguided belief. An excellent affirmation would be, "life always provides me with opportunity." Or "I am showered with gifts from the universe." Allow yourself to be open to the possibilities.

16

PUTTING IT ALL TOGETHER
ENERGETIC SEQUENCES FOR GUIDANCE, PROTECTION, AND CLARITY

Now that you recognize the power behind the practice with the tools to experience restorative yoga, the question still stands, "how do we put it all together?" The simple answer is: "it depends." How do you need to support yourself today? What is going to make you feel balanced? How much time are you allocating for your practice? Intention, breath, and postures are all part of the equation when putting together a sequence.

Tapping into what we need through intention is a major part of the practice. Having this self-awareness is like accessing a compass that we can use to feel balanced and whole. Each technique and posture can help us lean into our radiant presence by focusing on the energetic properties of a chakra, or through evoking a specific feeling—whether that corresponds physically or emotionally.

When we experience these shapes and methods, we can ask ourselves the following questions: is the posture grounding or buoyant? Open or introspective? Welcoming or cleansing? We all want the answers, but in reality, our experience will tell us what direction the intention is moving towards. The resources you've been offered in this book are suggestions based on someone else's experience, yet your involvement is all that truly matters. Getting curious about the postures will allow you to feel their potency and what qualities they bring out for you.

For example, if you work at a computer a lot and find yourself rounding forward, then backbends, shoulder, and chest openers are the remedy. The same focus can apply for anyone wanting to create more openness for love, forgiveness, and compassion on an energetic level. In this situation, rather than getting stuck practicing the asana that share a direct connection with the intention, consider how a range of different physical expressions can create an impact holistically. In this instance, releasing the hips will also benefit those who work on a computer after sitting for long periods, while those experiencing heartache may benefit from the emotional release associated with the hips. Exploring a varied practice will still support the intention while providing deeper insight into the inner workings of the entire system, rather than just its separate parts. One question some practitioners have is, "should my intention be physical or spiritual?"

The fear around having a purely physical intention is the idea that it dilutes the true essence of the practice. If this has crossed your mind, I have great news for you. The body-mind connection is very real and to take it one step further, the body-mind-spirit connection is also very real. If you are experiencing pain or restriction in a specific area, holding space to heal on a physical level will support the spirit. On the flip side, if we have a spiritual intention—like focusing on a specific chakra—it will result in the healing of the body. One might arrive on the mat with one intention but as time passes, that shifts and changes.

When I first set foot in a hatha yoga class, I thought I was just coming to condition my body, but over time, a deeper connection was made that romanced my spirit. Although this evolved over many years, intention can shift over the course of a single practice too. There have been many days that I've settled on my mat thinking that I need one focus, but what unfolds is very different. This illustrates the importance of remaining open and honest with ourselves. By staying vulnerable, we tune in to the subtle messages brought to the body, mind, and spirit meant to help us stay balanced.

Now that we have a clearer picture of intention, let's dig deeper into that question on timing. In a perfect world, we would be able to practice for 1 – 2 hours every day. When allocating that time becomes a challenge, we must recognize that every little bit counts. Even just 15 minutes can be a game-changer. So, do we jam as many postures into a 15-minute segment as possible, or practice just one or two postures?

My suggestion circles back to the intention of restorative yoga and the notion that time heals all wounds. To recap, staying in postures for longer periods of time allows us to shift deeper into a parasympathetic state and gives the mind enough time to unwind with the help of a meditative focus. Every restorative practice should be made up of these four elements: grounding, breath focus, posture(s), and relaxation (savasana). Grounding can be made up of pranayama or a meditation, including a body scan, while breath brings us the awareness of what space is created. The postures tell us where we can invite more relaxation, while savasana gives us room to let go. In the case of a 15-minute practice, the sequence may only incorporate one posture, but ticks all the other boxes as well.

Finally, you may be wondering why certain poses are strung together in a specific sequence. So, is there a specific order they have to go in? Although there's not an exact science when it comes to sequencing, it does follow basic principles, meaning that there is an art to putting the pieces together. Considering the first element is grounding, you start in postures that are the most relaxing or easeful. Examples of this might be savasana, seated for a pranayama or meditation, or a restorative posture that maximizes comfort, like a simple supported backbend or supported butterfly. Then, consider which following postures would be easy to transition into. For example, if you are lying down, it might make sense to practice another posture lying down.

Another key thought to consider: is my body ready for this next posture? For instance, some students find that warming up their spine with cat and cow before doing a supported child's pose is ideal. Others may appreciate practicing a twist before a backbend, while some prefer the opposite. With sequencing, it's less about what's "right" or "wrong" and more about what your body is asking for out of a sequence.

SEQUENCING AND TRANSITIONS

When creating a sequence, the question to ask yourself is "can I do this with ease?" Transitions can be just as blissful as the posture itself with the right mindset. Just as in life, there can be a tendency to rush to the "main event" rather than enjoy the ride. By sequencing and transitioning mindfully, it's an opportunity to enjoy every moment. Instead of rushing through to get to "the next thing," suddenly there are more occasions to be fully present. Even the parts in between can be a moving meditation when we stay connected to the experience through body and breath. To do this gracefully, there are a few points to consider.

The direction that you are facing can influence how easily you transition into and out of a posture. For instance, in some cases it makes sense to face "the back" of the mat and change the orientation so that less effort is used. For example, if you are down on your belly facing towards the front of the mat, doesn't it make sense to keep this same orientation if you flipped onto your back? Imagine the fuss to change the orientation, it'd be a full 180! Not to mention an awkward and clunky change. The more graceful and effortless the transition, the better, which may mean switching up the orientation.

Another step to consider is how to fill the moments in between postures. Before transitioning, a counterpose might be a welcomed addition to the sequence. A counterpose is defined as an asana that integrates the action of the previous pose. This can involve moving in the opposite direction—like extending the spine through a backbend after flexion in a forward fold—or returning to a neutral position. When a counterpose is practiced, it is also an invitation to experience how the previous posture affected the body, either in the tissues or through breath. Counterposes can be static or dynamic. Here are a few excellent examples:

Knees to Chest

As the name suggests, this counterpose allows for knees to draw in towards chest. It can be practiced from seated or lying down, after a backbend or with a twist—either between sides and/or afterwards.

From lying down, this posture can be static or dynamic. Dynamic options include rocking side to side, knee circles, or a variation known as "apanasana" or apana-releasing pose. Apana being the downward and outward flow of energy that releases what the body or energetic field no longer needs. To practice apanasana, pulse knees into chest. Exhaling as knees draw closer, inhaling to release the pressure.

Hip Movement

This is a choice designed for movement in the hip socket to assist as a counterpose after hip opening. Practiced with knees bent or legs straight, legs will move side to side. From lying down with knees bent, both knees move to one side, then the other, alternating with breath. Exhaling as knees release to one side, inhaling to lift up to center. With legs straight, typically the movement is quicker—and can be done sitting up or lying down—where the femur (upper leg bone) rotates externally and internally (outwards and inwards) rhythmically. Breathing stays long and steady.

Cat and Cow

A perfect posture to practice from all fours or seated, cat and cow uses dynamic spinal extension and flexion which can feel wonderful after practicing either action. Typically, spinal flexion—or cat—is performed on an exhale to lengthen tailbone down, round through the back, then release the head down, followed by an inhale for spinal extension—or cow—by lifting the tailbone, lowering the belly, and lifting the gaze. Practicing cat cow from seated has the same movements that initiate from the base of the spine that remain linked to breath. Cat cow—although usually dynamic—creates opportunities to pause as well. For instance, after a backbend it might feel intuitive to round through your back to practice cat and linger for a few extra cycles of breath.

Foot Pedaling

On all fours, lengthen one leg back behind you, plant the ball of your foot—draw your heel towards the mat. Lower knee back down. Switch sides. Keep alternating using your breath. Playing with inhaling or exhaling while extending and doing the opposite (inhaling or exhaling) when knee lowers down. Example of foot pedaling in the figure below.

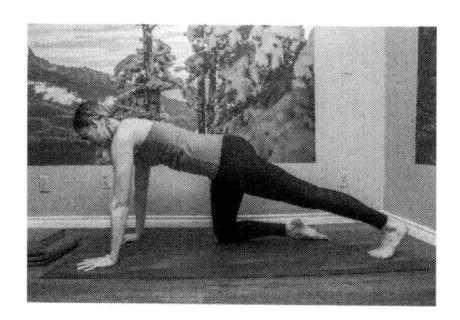

Fig. 16.1

Sufi Grind

With similar features to cat and cow, sufi grind is unique in that it allows for lateral (or side) flexion. Moving cyclically creates fluidity in the body—specifically for the spine—that can feel very nourishing. To practice from seated (or all fours), start making circles with your spine —inhaling as your heart and body shift forward, exhaling as it circles around back behind you. Use your breath to set the pace.

Hip Circles

From all fours, hip circles have a similar benefit to sufi grind in terms of fluidity but foster this quality in the pelvis rather than the spine. For those who feel "stuck" or stagnant in this area, hip circles can feel very freeing. Take a wider stance on all fours (hands slightly ahead of shoulders), start circling hips—inhaling as hips swing forward, exhaling as they circle back towards heels. These circles can be as small or as big as you want. Move in one direction for 3 – 10 cycles of breath, then switch.

Deconstructive Rest Pose

This can feel soothing for the lower back. Done statically, deconstructive rest pose allows for internal rotation of the thighs. This internal rotation allows the back of the pelvis to widen, creating more space for the sacroiliac joints which connect the sacrum (the flat bone at the base of your spine) to the ilia (hip bone). To practice deconstructive rest pose, have knees bent and step feet wide on your mat. Let knees relax inwards so they rest against one another.

Finally, breath will always support you through transitions. Instead of rushing to the next posture, use the time to appreciate how breath moves through your body. Notice the cycle of inhalations and exhalations that stay with us, day in and day out, until the last breath we take. So much gratitude can be drawn from the act of breathing—happening with or without our knowledge. Seeing the beauty in these transitions might make us realize how those "in-between" moments in our lives hold a special place in our heart too.

EXAMPLE SEQUENCES

Below are full-length examples of sequences paired with potential intentions to draw inspiration from. Feel empowered to experiment, mix-and-match, and explore which sequences work best for you.

LETTING GO OF EMOTIONAL WEIGHT: 1 HOUR

- Seated in sukhasana: vishama vritti pranayama for 5 minutes

- Supported bound angle with a bolster 15 minutes

- Supported twist with a bolster 7 minutes each side—3x clearing breaths before transitioning out of each side (1 minute in between to transition)

- Supported heart opening bridge for 10 minutes (set up and transition out 5 minutes)

- Savasana 10 minutes

FREEDOM TO BREATHE: FEELING YOUR FULL BREATH POTENTIAL 1 HR 15 MINS

- Legs up the wall practice dirga pranayama 10 minutes

- Side lying release 8 minutes each side (4 minutes between sides for transition)

- Simple supported backbend—thoracic fish variation 10 minutes

- Forward fold 8 minutes

- Simple supported backbend with bolster 10 minutes (2 minute transition afterwards)

- Savasana 15 minutes

BLISSFUL HIPS: LIBERATING THE AREA AROUND THE PELVIS 1 HR

- Supported bound angle (no bolster) 15 minutes—practice 10 rounds of brahmari while in the posture before settling into stillness

- Reclined side lying release 7 minutes each side (1 minute transition in between sides)

- Supported seated angle 8 minutes (2 minutes for counterposing/transition)

- Supported bridge 9 minutes (a minute or two to transition)

- Savasana 10 minutes

CREATING SPACE FOR INNER STRENGTH

- Ujayyi breathing in sukhasana 8 minutes

- Cat/cow 2 minutes

- Supported sphynx 8 minutes (2 minutes for counterpose and transition)

- Supported Child's Pose 7 minutes (3 minutes for counterpose and transition)

- Supported Hero's Pose 7 minutes (3 minutes for counterpose and transition)

- Legs up the wall with dirga pranayama 10 minutes

- Savasana 10 minutes

EPILOGUE

While I was writing this book, I wondered how I would be "wrapping it up." I thought to myself, "everything that needs to be said has already been said." Boy, was I wrong! I was about a month away from launching my book when the devastating events related to COVID-19 hit my community along with the rest of the world. Everything came to a standstill. As a collective consciousness, stress levels went through the roof with the level of uncertainty. It seemed like the rug had been pulled out from under everyone's first chakra, including my own. I closed the studio that I had put my heart and soul into, unsure of when we'd be able to operate again.

There wasn't a single person I knew who hadn't been impacted by this severe event in some way. The shared intensity reminded me of a card from the Tarot deck known as "The Tower"—often associated with fury, destruction, and peril. In the week that everything plummeted out of control, I did a tarot reading for myself and this card came up in a position that signifies "guidance." I laughed when I saw it. "How could this be my guidance card?" I found myself asking with an eye roll.

EPILOGUE

I was in the midst of riding a wave of ambiguity—that played out sometimes hour by hour—doing my best to stay centered as everything around me fell apart. I tried to continue reading a wonderful book about manifesting and attracting, but my knee-jerk reaction defaulted to anger, "how can we attract what we want when everything is going to shit?!" It all felt like a lie. Even though these were the principles I believed in whole-heartedly, I still found that doubt snuck in the minute it had the chance.

Everyone falls off "the path" sometimes. Life circumstances can hit hard. Mistakes happen. Being human is never perfect. All we can ask is that we are able to pull ourselves up by our spiritual bootstraps and recognize that this too, is part of the process. Through our yoga practice, we can meet ourselves where we are, rather than where our ego thinks we're "meant to be." We then become aware that the messages and teachings we experience on the mat are also reflected in the experiences of life. In the tough moments, each of us can choose to acknowledge the wisdom we've always known deep in our hearts. The knowledge that we are loved, guided, and held so that we may move in the right direction—even when it doesn't seem like it.

This seemingly basic spiritual tenet is likely one of the toughest to fully digest as it requires us to accept, surrender, and trust. The more that we can lean into these qualities in our practice, the easier it will be to embrace them in real life when we're thrown a curve ball. So, what are you waiting for? Now is the time to begin again. We start by committing to the guidelines of Restorative Yoga with a Capital "R." This includes focusing on subtle sensations, staying in postures for longer periods of time, using an abundance of props, and holding space for stillness.

Embracing this idea of slowing down can be met through challenging a rebellious mind with a point of focus (dharana). Rising to this challenge asks us to look at what we can let go of, especially any expectations that feel heavy, like what we "should" look like, do, or feel. If we are seeking the "perfect moment" to find peace, then peace will never come and we'll always be one distraction away from bliss. Instead, there's an opportunity to explore the perfection of the moment without trying to control the outcome, and that's when true bliss breaks though. Beyond the taming of the mind, there's the journey of aligning ourselves energetically. The chakra system can be used like a compass, pinpointing areas that feel "stuck" or stagnant and clarifying what feels open or in sync with the cosmic flow. This subtle energetic map is easier to access when we "tune in" on a physical and mental level by practicing deep relaxation.

Beyond the clarity and resilience that comes with profound relaxation, there's one final message that surfaces with sincere practice: the realization that we are already enough. These gifts are already inside of us. We don't have to go out searching for answers or try to find the light that feels like it's lost—we are already that light, we are already all that we seek. Yet every now and then, we forget. Our yoga and mindfulness practices can help us remember by peeling back the layers that don't resonate with our true self so that we return to that brilliance and grace. Like wiping off a clouded mirror, sometimes we need to do a little spiritual cleaning of our own to see everything from a fresh lens.

After tossing my book down and seeing my emotions grab hold of me, I recognized the need to look at this situation through a fresh lens. After all, these teachings were part of my truth! I knew they had been a beacon in my darkest times and would continue to follow me until my last breath. With clearer insight, it became blatantly obvious that this anger, doubt, and despair had an unmistakable energetic imprint —The Tower was out in full force! However, just as we face each circumstance in life, each card always has two outcomes. The other interpretation leans into the power of transformation, asking us to break down the old to welcome the new with unwavering faith. This process of renewal illustrates how the difficult moments in life ask each of us to step into the unknown and by taking this leap of faith,

EPILOGUE

we open ourselves up to new possibilities that we'd never even imagined.

That old job, or relationship, or whatever life circumstance it may be, can shift, change, or be destroyed altogether for something bigger and more beautiful than we ever could've thought possible. If anything, these experiences are a wake-up call to celebrate the tenacity of the human spirit. Even when parts of ourselves feel panicked, angry, exhausted or sad, the strength inside of us remains unshaken. Rather than dwell in the mundane, we are meant to be stirred up so that we can be reminded of what is truly important, while moving towards our best and brightest selves. Instead of the world happening to us, it's possible that it is happening for us. Just maybe, everything is unfolding exactly how it should.

ABOUT THE AUTHOR

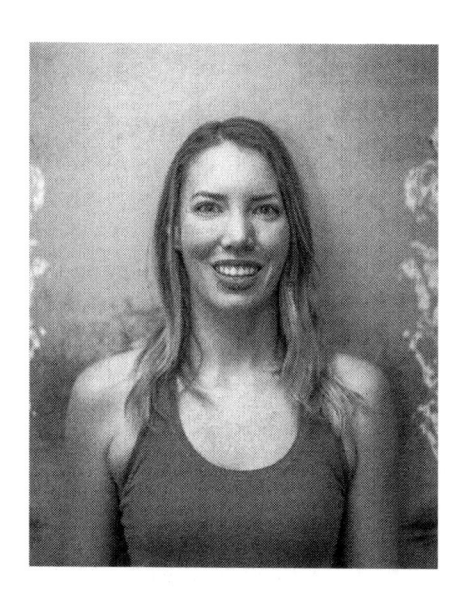

Emily Kane is an ERYT-500, BKin, Reiki Master Teacher, and Thai Medicine Practitioner. Her therapeutic style seeks to hold space in a truly profound way with a refreshing holistic approach. Emily has helped people from around the world come back to themselves through yoga and energetic work. Her articles have been featured in major publications including Elephant Journal and Wanderlust.

ABOUT THE AUTHOR

She teaches public classes, yoga teacher trainings, workshops, and reiki certifications at her studio in Whistler BC and worldwide.

Find the author at @emilykaneyoga and her studio @yogacarawhistler

Websites: www.emilykaneyoga.com and www.whistleryogacara.com

REFERENCES

"The deeper philosophical teachings from this book are based on interpretations of the ancient wisdom that includes but is not limited to the Vedas, Upanishads, Yoga Sutras, and Hatha Yoga Pradipika. These teachings are the roots of yoga, Hinduism, and can act as an inspiration to all, regardless of what faith one follows."

Abraham, S. B., Rubino, D., Sinaii, N., Ramsey, S., & Nieman, L. K. (2013). Cortisol, obesity, and the metabolic syndrome: A cross-sectional study of obese subjects and review of the literature. *Obesity (Silver Spring, Md.)*, *21*(1), E105-E117. https://doi.org/10.1002/oby.20083

Asadollahi, T., Khakpour, S., Ahmadi, F., Seyedeh, L., Tahami, Matoo, S., & Bermas, H. (2015). Effectiveness of mindfulness training and dietary regime on weight loss in obese people. *Journal of Medicine and Life*, *8*(Special Issue 4), 114-124. Retrieved from http://www.medandlife.ro

Brigham Young University - Idaho. (2013). *Organization of the nervous system* [Figure]. Retrieved from https://content.byui.edu/file/

REFERENCES

a236934c-3c60-4fe9-90aa-d343b3e3a640/1/module10/readings/org_nerve_system.html

Brown, B. (2010). *The gifts of imperfection: Let go of who you think you're supposed to be and embrace who you are.* Center City, MN: Hazelden.

CK-12 Foundation. (n.d.). *Levels of organization of the nervous system* [Figure]. Retrieved from https://www.ck12.org/c/biology/peripheral-nervous-system/lesson/The-Peripheral-Nervous-System-Advanced-BIO-ADV/

Daneshmandi, H., Choobineh, A., Ghaem, H., & Karimi, M. (2017). Adverse effects of prolonged sitting behavior on the general health of office workers. *Journal of Lifestyle Medicine, 7*(2), 69-75. https://doi.org/10.15280/jlm.2017.7.2.69

Ezrin, S. (2019). This 7-pose home practice will help you close (yes, close) your heart after grief. Retrieved from http://www.yogajournal.com/practice/yoga-for-grief

Gooley, J. J., Chamberlain, K., Smith, K. A., Khalsa, S. B., Rajaratnam, S. M., Van Reen, E., . . . Lockley, S. W. (2011). Exposure to room light before bedtime suppresses melatonin onset and shortens melatonin duration in humans. *Journal of Clinical Endocrinology and Metabolism, 96*(3), E463-472. https://doi.org/10.1210/jc.2010-2098

Guardian News. (2019, October 30). Barack Obama takes on 'woke' call-out culture: 'That's not activism' [Video file]. Retrieved from http://www.youtube.com/watch?v=qaHLd8de6nM

Hargrove, T. (2009). The SAID principle. Retrieved from http://www.bettermovement.org/blog/2009/0110111

Hay, L. [Louise Hay]. (2017, October 27). Louise Hay's top 10 rules for success [Video file]. Retrieved from https://www.youtube.com/watch?v=yie6ynC69R8

Hayduke, D., & Nye, A. (2019). C-60 The efficacy of weighted blankets for quantity and quality of sleep in autism spectrum disorder: A meta-analysis. *Archives of Clinical Neuropsychology, 34*(6), 1089. https://doi.org/10.1093/arclin/acz034.222

Hormone Health Network. (2018). Stress and your health | Endocrine Society. Retrieved from https://www.hormone.org/your-health-and-hormones/stress-and-your-health

Hugh-Jones, S., & Smith, P. K. (1999). Self-reports of short- and long-term effects of bullying on children who stammer. *British Journal of Educational Psychology, 69*(2), 141-158. https://doi.org/10.1348/000709999157626

Ingraham, P. (2017). IT band stretching does not work. Retrieved from http://www.painscience.com/articles/iliotibial-band-syndrome-stretch.php

Kaivalya, A., & van der Kooij, A. (2010). *Myths of the asanas: The stories at the heart of the yoga tradition.* San Rafael, CA: Mandala Publishing.

Kizirian, A. (n.d.). *Functional organization of the PNS* [Figure]. Retrieved from https://antranik.org/visceral-sensory-neurons-and-referred-pain/

Lagopoulos, J., Xu, J., Rasmussen, I., Vik, A., Malhi, G. S., Eliassen, C. F., . . . Ellingsen, Ø. (2009). Increased theta and alpha EEG activity during nondirective meditation. *Journal of Alternative and Complementary Medicine, 15*(11), 1187-1192. https://doi.org/10.1089/acm.2009.0113

Lasater, J. H. (2009). *Yogabody: Anatomy, kinesiology, and asana.* Berkeley, CA: Rodmell Press.

Lee, D.-E., Seo, S.-M., Woo, H.-S., & Won, S.-Y. (2018). Analysis of body imbalance in various writing sitting postures using sitting pressure measurement. *Journal of Physical Therapy Science, 30*(2), 343-346. https://doi.org/10.1589/jpts.30.343

Leelarungrayub, D., Pothongsunun, P., Yankai, A., & Pratanaphon, S. (2009). Acute clinical benefits of chest wall-stretching exercise on

REFERENCES

expired tidal volume, dyspnea and chest expansion in a patient with chronic obstructive pulmonary disease: A single case study. *Journal of Bodywork and Movement Therapies, 13*(4), 338-343. https://doi.org/10.1016/j.jbmt.2008.11.004

Liao, D., Rodríguez-Colón, S. M., He, F., & Bixler, E. O. (2014). Childhood obesity and autonomic dysfunction: Risk for cardiac morbidity and mortality. *Current Treatment Options in Cardiovascular Medicine, 16*(10), 342. https://doi.org/10.1007/s11936-014-0342-1

Lumen Learning. (n.d.). Functions of the autonomic nervous system. Retrieved from http://courses.lumenlearning.com/boundless-ap/chapter/functions-of-the-autonomic-nervous-system/

Lumpkin, N., & Khalsa, J. K. (n.d.). The heart chakra. Retrieved from http://www.3ho.org/heart-chakra

Lurati, A. R. (2018). Health issues and injury risks associated with prolonged sitting and sedentary lifestyles. *Workplace Health & Safety, 66*(6), 285-290. https://doi.org/10.1177/2165079917737558

Marieb, E. N., & Hoehn, K. N. (2012). *Human anatomy & physiology* (8th ed., Florida ed.). Boston, MA: Pearson Learning Solutions.

Mayo Clinic. (2019). Pinched nerve. Retrieved from http://www.mayoclinic.org/diseases-conditions/pinched-nerve/symptoms-causes/syc-20354746

McCorry, L. K. (2007). Physiology of the autonomic nervous system. *American Journal of Pharmaceutical Education, 71*(4), 78. Retrieved from https://www.ncbi.nlm.nih.gov/pmc/articles/PMC1959222/

McCraty, R. (2015). *Science of the heart: Exploring the role of the heart in human performance* (Vol. 2). Boulder Creek, CA: HeartMath Institute.

Moreno-Smith, M., Lutgendorf, S. K., & Sood, A. K. (2010). Impact of stress on cancer metastasis. *Future Oncology (London, England), 6*(12), 1863-1881. https://doi.org/10.2217/fon.10.142

Myss, C. (2004). *Invisible acts of power: Channeling grace in your everyday life*. New York, NY: Free Press.

Nall, R. (2019). What to know about nitric oxide supplements. *Medically reviewed by Zara Risoldi Cochrane, Pharm.D., M.S., FASCP. Medical News Today*. Retrieved from https://www.medicalnewstoday.com/articles/326381

Perry, P. (2018). Can you really pick up on good and bad 'vibes'? Yes, suggests new research. Retrieved from https://bigthink.com/sensing-vibes

Qualitative Reasoning Group Northwestern University. (n.d.). Propulsion: Every action has an equal and opposite reaction? Retrieved from http://www.qrg.northwestern.edu/projects/vss/docs/propulsion/2-every-action-has-an-equal-and-opposite.html

Rabago, D., & Zgierska, A. (2009). Saline nasal irrigation for upper respiratory conditions. *American Family Physician, 80*(10), 1117-1119. Retrieved from https://www.aafp.org/journals/afp.html

Reynolds, J. L. (2019). Having empathy and being an empath: What's the difference? Retrieved from http://www.psychologytoday.com/ca/blog/human-kind/201901/having-empathy-and-being-empath-what-s-the-difference

Salmon, G., James, A., & Smith, D. M. (1998). Bullying in schools: Self reported anxiety, depression, and self esteem in secondary school children. *British Medical Journal, 317*(7163), 924-925. https://doi.org/10.1136/bmj.317.7163.924

Santos-Longhurst, A. (2019). What are glands in the body? *Medically reviewed by Alana Biggers, M.D., MPH. Healthline*. Retrieved from http://www.healthline.com/health/what-are-glands#problems-with-glands

Saoji, A. A., Raghavendra, B. R., & Manjunath, N. K. (2019). Effects of yogic breath regulation: A narrative review of scientific evidence. *Journal of Ayurveda and Integrative Medicine, 10*(1), 50-58. https://doi.org/10.1016/j.jaim.2017.07.008

REFERENCES

Sapolsky, R. M. (1992). *Stress, the aging brain, and the mechanisms of neuron death.* Cambridge, MA: The MIT Press.

Sapolsky, R. M., Krey, L. C., & McEwen, B. S. (1986). The neuroendocrinology of stress and aging: The glucocorticoid cascade hypothesis. *Endocrine Reviews, 7*(3), 284-301. https://doi.org/10.1210/edrv-7-3-284

Shaffer, J. (2016). Neuroplasticity and clinical practice: Building brain power for health. *Frontiers in Psychology, 7,* 1118. https://doi.org/10.3389/fpsyg.2016.01118

Specktor, B. (2018). Why are pregnant women told to sleep on their left side? Retrieved from http://www.livescience.com/63375-why-sleep-left-side-pregnant.html

Tan, D. X., Xu, B., Zhou, X., & Reiter, R. J. (2018). Pineal calcification, melatonin production, aging, associated health consequences and rejuvenation of the pineal gland. *Molecules, 23*(2), 301. https://doi.org/10.3390/molecules23020301

Weitzberg, E., & Lundberg, J. O. (2002). Humming greatly increases nasal nitric oxide. *American Journal of Respiratory and Critical Care Medicine, 166*(2), 144-145. https://doi.org/10.1164/rccm.200202-138BC

Wolff, P., & Shepard, J. (2013). Causation, touch, and the perception of force. In B. H. Ross (Ed.), *Psychology of Learning and Motivation* (Vol. 58, pp. 167-202). Cambridge, MA: Academic Press.

Copyright © 2020 Emily Kane

The Energy & Art of Restorative Yoga

All rights reserved.

Contributors:

Primary Editor: Helena Gerrelli

Additional Editors: Ross Hacquebard, Kevin Day, Maeve Jones, Ingrid Vanderwey

Book Coach: Mike Skrypnek

Cover Photo: Justa Jeskova

Photos in Book: Jeremy Allen

Diagrams: Juan Villegas

Reference Organization: Jess Hewitt

Formatting: Fallon Publishing

No part of this publication may be reproduced, stored in a retrieval system or transmitted in any form or by any means, electronic, mechanical, photocopying, recording or otherwise, without prior permission. For information about permissions or about discounts for bulk orders or to book an event with the author or his colleagues or any other matter, please write to the author.

Disclaimer: This book contains the opinions and ideas of the author and is offered for information purposes only.

The author and publisher specifically disclaim responsibility for any liability loss or risk personal or otherwise, which is incurred as a consequence, directly or indirectly, of the use and application of any of the contents of this book.